STARVING THE WOLF

A Victory Over Lupus

Transformative Strategies for
Reclaiming Health & Vitality

Karen Quiros, CHC

Positive Psychology Practitioner, Licensed Nurse

Over 25 Years Lupus Free!

Cover design by MindtheMargins, LLC
Cover image by iStock mirceax
Wolf icon courtesy of Clker-Free-Vector-Images
All other icons courtesy of Freepik.com

ISBN: 979-8-9895349-0-6 (digital online)
ISBN: 979-8-9895349-1-3 (paperback)
ISBN: 979-8-9895349-2-0 (hardcover)

Printed in USA

For permissions, inquiries, or further information,
please contact: karen@balwell.com

TABLE OF CONTENTS

DEDICATION

For all the Lupus Warriors, Daring Pioneers, and Rising Phoenixes

More than just a chronicle of lupus and endometriosis, this book, born from my healing journey, is dedicated to you. It acts as a mirror, reflecting your struggles—a portrayal of the unseen battles you face daily, the quiet victories hidden in the fog of fatigue, and your indomitable spirit that gracefully confronts pain without giving in.

Within these pages, you won't discover magic spells or miraculous drugs but something more potent: a reminder of the latent power residing within you. The greatest healer does not dwell in a pill or procedure but in the silent wisdom humming beneath the surface of their existence.

Warriors, embrace the quiet strength and resilience woven into the essence of your being. Trust your intuition—it's the guiding whisper through the mist of pain, an inner compass leading you toward paths of solace and healing.

Starving the Wolf stands as a beacon, not a blueprint. It attests to the significance of listening to your inner wisdom and mind and body, honoring its rhythms and nurturing its whispers with self-compassion and steadfast belief.

May this book serve as a reminder that even in the darkest nights, the stars still shine, and within you, a universe of healing light awaits. May its words soothe your weary soul and fuel your flickering flame.

Go forth, pioneers. Dance with the unknown, and never forget: You are not alone. You are not broken. You are healing.

And may the strength you find in healing inspire others on the same journey.

In solidarity and unwavering belief,
Karen

DISCLAIMER

Please note that the information provided in this book is intended for educational and informational purposes only. The content presented here is based on my personal research, experiences, and observations. The healing suggestions and tips included in this book may vary in their level of orthodoxy, ranging from conventional to unconventional. The author and publisher make no representations or warranties with respect to the accuracy, applicability, or completeness of the contents of this book.

It is essential to understand that every individual's health circumstances are unique, and what works for one person may not work for another. Therefore, *it is crucial to consult with your medical healthcare practitioner or a qualified healthcare professional before implementing any suggestions or making changes to your current treatment plan.* Your healthcare provider is the best equipped person to evaluate your specific health conditions, medical history, and individual needs, and provide personalized guidance and recommendations.

While I have made efforts to ensure the accuracy and reliability of the information provided, I cannot guarantee the completeness, timeliness, or effectiveness of the healing suggestions in this book. Furthermore, I make no promises or claims regarding your healing or the outcomes that may result from implementing any of the suggestions.

It is also important to note that any healing journey, including self-healing, is a multifaceted process that may require a combination of approaches, including professional medical care, lifestyle changes, and emotional well-being practices. The suggestions in this book are not intended to replace professional medical advice, diagnosis, or treatment. Always seek the guidance of qualified healthcare professionals regarding any medical conditions or concerns you may have.

By reading and utilizing the information in this book, you acknowledge and accept that you are solely responsible for your health decisions and actions. The author, publisher, and affiliated parties disclaim any liability for any direct, indirect, consequential, or incidental damages or losses that may arise from the use or misuse of the information provided in this book.

It is recommended to use your judgment, proceed with caution, and make informed choices that align with your individual circumstances and in consultation with appropriate healthcare professionals.

ACKNOWLEDGMENTS

Starving the Wolf was sparked by an unwavering belief in healing for myself and others walking the path of chronic illness. I am eternally grateful to everyone who shared this belief and helped guide my words to their destination.

To my husband and sons: Thank you for being my rock throughout the writing process. When late nights blurred into early mornings and research papers engulfed the dining room table instead of dinner, your unwavering support became my anchor. Gratitude fills my heart for the love and patience you extended. Your understanding, encouragement, hugs, and cups of tea were the steadying force that helped me navigate the challenges of this journey. During the chaos, you remained my haven, reminding me that the essence of family is what truly sustains.

To my friends, my confidants and sounding boards: Thank you for listening to my ideas, offering encouragement, and providing a welcome escape from the solitary world of writing. Your unwavering friendship and understanding were essential in keeping me grounded and focused.

To my clients, the courageous pioneers: Your stories fueled my passion. Your journeys mirrored my own—each struggle and triumph is a testament to the transformative power of healing. Thank you for trusting me and inspiring me to finish writing this book.

To the doctors who gave me a limited life expectancy: You inadvertently fueled my determination. Your skepticism became my fire, and proving the prognosis wrong became my driving force. You challenged me to rewrite my destiny, and I am thankful for that.

To the dedicated editors and proofreaders: Your patience and meticulous eyes transformed my rough draft into a cohesive and polished work. Your expertise and dedication are deeply appreciated. Your collective commitment to excellence challenged me to refine my thoughts and articulate my ideas with precision.

To the visionary artist and layout architect: Your creative eye transformed the essence of *Starving the Wolf* into a stunning visual experience, from the captivating cover that sparks curiosity to the elegant interior design that guides readers through my journey. Thank you for being the artistic anchor that welcomed my vision and brought my words to life on the page.

And to those who inquired about the book's progress: Your genuine interest provided a welcome nudge forward, even when progress felt slow. Your reminders of the profound impact this book holds were instrumental in keeping the journey alive.

Together, you have all contributed to this profoundly rewarding experience, and for that, I am forever grateful.

With heartfelt gratitude and appreciation,
Karen

Visit **www.starvingthewolf.com**
and subscribe to receive exclusive updates.

You'll have early access to
new content, events, and projects
that expand on the insights shared in this book.

Never be bullied into silence.
Never allow yourself to be made a victim.
Accept no one's definition of your life; define yourself.

—Harvey Fierstein

He who has a why to live
can bear almost any how.

—Friedrich Nietzsche

PREFACE

In the depths of my struggle with systemic and discoid lupus, I embarked on a courageous journey to reclaim my health and defy the limitations imposed by this mysterious disease. I knew the path to healing would not be paved by hope or wishful thinking; it required unwavering determination and an insatiable thirst for knowledge. With each passing day, I delved into the vast realm of lupus, voraciously devouring information, dissecting scientific studies, and meticulously analyzing my symptoms.

Lupus, a labyrinth of mysteries, manifests differently in each individual it dares to touch. Yet, amid the complexity, I found a glimmer of certainty—an unwavering belief that reducing inflammation was the key to unlocking recovery. I understood that inflammation, like an invisible saboteur, was insidiously fueling the fires of pain, fatigue, and despair within my body. It was the common thread that wove together the myriad triggers: my thoughts, my diets, my actions, and the intangible that surrounds us.

As I set forth on this expedition, I yearned to heal myself and illuminate a path for others trapped in the clutches of lupus. I implore you, dear reader, if there is but one message to be gleaned from the following pages, let it be this: embrace the quest to prevent and tame inflammation within you. In dismantling the stronghold of inflammation, we lay the foundation upon which the cure shall arise. So, I invite you to embark upon this odyssey with me to forge a pact with knowledge, determination, and the unwavering belief that we have the power to overcome. Let us weave our stories into a tapestry of triumph over adversity, and together, let us conquer lupus.

GUIDED BY PASSION AND PURPOSE

During my lupus healing journey, a pivotal moment reshaped my understanding of life and purpose. The car I was a passenger in hit a tree. The horn blared, and forces that felt like a vacuum yanked me out of my seat, pulling me up and away from the wreckage. As I ascended, the sound of the horn grew distant, and I knew I was leaving this world. In those moments, the boundary between life and something beyond blurred. It was a profound spiritual experience that transcended the physical realm. It was in that surreal space that I heard direction: "It is not your time. You must return to ease the suffering of others."

I wondered, how I could help others when I myself was dying, when doctors had just told me that I only had five to seven years to live? How could I ease others' suffering when I was so sick? The answer remained a mystery, lost in the haze of my impending return. When I came back to our physical world, I found myself in the emergency room, surrounded by medical professionals cutting off my favorite denim jacket. The world rushed back in a whirl of fluorescent lights, pain, and anxious voices. I had returned from the brink, but the message of purpose lingered.

Over the next decade, higher guidance unfolded, leading me down uncharted paths, and I healed. Some may call it divine guidance, destiny, fate, or extraordinary healing, but it is all the same miraculous force that transcends science and medicine to heal body, mind, and spirit—a oneness that connects us all. Through quiet reflection, meditation, and whispers of inner wisdom, I gained clarity and direction on my healing journey and purpose. I explored fields of study, embraced holistic practices, nourished my body, and shared my insights with others.

This book is a testament to that guidance—a journey of self-discovery, faith, and the profound connection we all have. I hope to ease your suffering and inspire you to heal yourself.

Lupus and endometriosis had taken their toll on me, but desperation led me to search for answers beyond conventional medicine. My quest for healing had taken on a spiritual dimension. Each morning, I meditated with a clear intention: to gain clarity and direction. To my amazement, I began to receive subtle and profound guidance during meditation. I received insights, sometimes like gentle nudges, other times like vivid visions or startling shouts, but always with clarity and purpose. Most times, I embraced these instructions with an open heart and mind.

When I followed this guidance, my health steadily improved. It nudged me to explore new fields of study, delve into plant medicine and energy healing, and adjust my diet. I acted on it all, driven by a passion for healing. Some days, the guidance was as simple as stepping outside to embrace the sun's warmth; others, it led me to take up a course of study. However, I also experienced moments of resistance, where I would ignore the guidance. These were the times when my healing would stall, a stark reminder that the guidance I received was not to be taken lightly. It was a gift, and to neglect it was to thwart my progress.

Starving the Wolf shares the outcomes of the guidance I received and the actions I took during my decade-long quest for healing from lupus and endometriosis. While my path was shaped by these specific challenges, the principles and insights I gained are universal. These general health-promoting tips can inspire healing and be embraced by anyone, regardless of their circumstances.

Healing knows no boundaries. It is an inclusive, compassionate force that offers its wisdom to all who seek it. I invite you to explore this force, embrace your inner wisdom, and remain open to the belief that you can heal and thrive. We all deserve to heal. I encourage you to walk this path with an open heart and mind, take what feels right, and leave the rest.

Finally, it's important to note that believing in a divine presence is not a prerequisite for finding healing. Instead, my references to the subject are meant as a heartfelt sharing of the tips and insights I've gained through the guidance I received. These insights are intended to ease suffering and promote overall well-being. Healing journeys come in various forms, and this book serves as a guidepost for those on a quest for a healthier and more fulfilling life.

INTRODUCTION

In the realm of healing, it can feel overwhelming to navigate through the abundance of conflicting information that now exists. For every study supporting the pros of a particular approach, you can easily find just as many advocating for the cons. Amid this sea of information, it's important to remember that you hold the power to decide what feels right for your own well-being. Trusting your intuition becomes a guiding light on this journey.

We are created with the ability to heal. Give your being the attention it needs, and it will flourish. Discovering what you need is a process with lessons in self-reliance, patience, and relentlessness. As you embark on your path to healing, remain open to learning and expanding your knowledge. Engage in thorough research, exploring different perspectives and approaches. Seek out experts in the field and ask them questions that resonate with your concerns. Remember that your body and your experiences are unique, and what works for one person may not work for another.

Ultimately, trust in your ability to make the right decisions for your body. You possess an innate wisdom that connects you to your own needs and desires. Listen closely to the whispers of your soul, for it can serve as a reliable compass, leading you toward the healing modalities that align with your divine self.

Above all, approach this journey with self-compassion and patience. Healing is not a linear process, and there may be setbacks along the way. Embrace the understanding that your body and mind are resilient, capable of transformation and renewal. Trust that you have the strength to adapt and adjust as needed, making informed choices that support your healing and well-being. Remember, you are the author of your healing story. Embrace your individuality, and trust your own wisdom. By combining intuition, research, expert guidance, and self-trust, you pave the way for a healing journey that is uniquely yours.

Please use this book as a starting point for your healing. I have written just enough on various topics to spark your interest, so that you can explore a topic on your own and see if it's something you'd like to include in your healing toolbox. Most of the individual topics in this book could fill the pages of a whole other book! I've tried to keep them concise, friendly, and actionable so that you can easily implement them and see if they feel right to you. Remember, love heals all, it really does, especially self-love.

Self-reliance and meticulous research are the cornerstones of this book's ethos. Self-reliance is our compass as we navigate the vast landscape of solutions, while research is our guide. Having walked this path myself, I can't emphasize enough the importance of preparation before embracing any alternative treatment. Whenever I encountered a new remedy that piqued my interest, my first step was always to conduct in-depth research. Consulting books, articles, and the firsthand experiences of others became my norm.

The next crucial step was to confer with my physicians. Throughout my journey, I was fortunate to curate a medical team that genuinely appreciated my commitment to self-healing and was open to discussing nontraditional treatments. Their insights and respect for my healing choices ensured that I was on a trajectory that was not only aligned with my beliefs but also safe for me. Their guidance enabled me to weigh the pros and cons adeptly, ensuring that I made decisions that prioritized my well-being. If there's one biggest piece of advice I'd give, it's to ensure that you have a supportive team.

While alternative paths can offer transformative experiences, not all that glitters is gold. Some treatments, masked under the guise of healing, can be scams or dangerous in other ways. Look for red flags like unrealistic promises, vast cure-all claims unsupported by science, exorbitant prices with pushy upfront payments, and practitioners lacking transparency or proper credentials. If a practitioner evades questions, resorts to fearmongering, or isn't forthcoming about their method's risks and side effects, take a step back and reconsider.

For those exploring alternative healers, it's essential to:

- Inquire about their credentials and training
- Seek reviews and firsthand accounts from others
- Delve into scientific studies or historical evidence backing their methods
- Demand a thorough explanation of their technique
- Ensure you're at ease with the practitioner

Balancing self-reliance with informed knowledge can be empowering. It can lead to finding the best solutions for one's unique health journey. Health is an invaluable treasure. Approaching each alternative avenue with curiosity, caution, and critical thinking will empower you to make decisions that genuinely resonate with your healing journey.

 ## My Lupus Journey

My experience with lupus was daunting, but I decided early on that my only option was to heal.

Over 35 years ago from the date I write this, after months of debilitating pain, exhaustion, fevers, hives, doctor visits, hospital stays, and a skin biopsy, I was branded with the diagnosis of systemic lupus erythematosus and discoid lupus, and was casually given five to seven years to live. I was told there wasn't a cure, and that there wasn't anything the medical community could do for me other than ease the symptoms. In addition to a long list of medications, I was referred to physical therapy and a lupus patient support group. My world came crashing down, and I felt lost and alone. The experts told me that death was imminent. They gave my life a rapidly approaching expiration date, even though I was only in my mid-twenties.

After a few months of following doctors' orders, I determined that the medications were not working for me because I was feeling much sicker. As my symptoms worsened, I turned to my faith in my ability to make my own best decisions. I decided to abandon the prescribed methods and try to find a cure on my own. I could not and would not live in misery and accept that I would die in my thirties. The doctors, understandably, told me I was making a huge mistake. Many in my family didn't support my decision either. But a death sentence is a call to action, not a time for retreat. Lupus was my teacher, and my faith was my guide.

I questioned and researched everything, leaving no stone unturned. I started with the assumption that anything could have triggered the deterioration of my immune system. I knew that if I could restore it, it would function optimally again. The energy of my belief fueled my healing. There were setbacks and suffering, but my faith never wavered. As I set forth on my healing journey, I recognized that I could no longer sustain lupus with the same beliefs, emotions, diet, or thoughts that had fueled its existence. Instead, I deliberately deprived lupus of the sustenance it required to persist. I came to call this "starving the wolf," which is where the title of this book comes from.

Today, and for the past 27-plus years, I live lupus-free. I am healed. I say 27-plus years because I restored my health before 1994, when I gave birth to my first child. Before attempting to get pregnant via in vitro fertilization, my OB/GYN doctor was concerned that pregnancy would exacerbate the disease and that I would no longer be in remission. I respected but graciously rejected their concern, because I knew I had healed. Doctors questioned and cautioned me during each of my visits. After giving birth, the doctors said I was lucky but shouldn't consider getting pregnant again because I might not be lucky a second time, that I should be appreciative of my healthy child but not take that risk again. Seven years later I gave birth to another healthy baby boy.

My health in the years that followed greatly improved, except for endometriosis and setbacks from abdominal adhesion surgeries. Through it all, my lupus blood markers and symptoms never returned. I knew that I had healed myself of lupus.

I was frustrated that I couldn't change my medical records to reflect that I was now healthy; frustrated that the medical community denied lupus could be cured. I lost faith in the system. Even though I *knew* I was healed, I still had to carry the label of disease on my medical records. I refused to accept the label. It's a system that relies on lab results to label a disease, but disregards lab results when they show no disease. Disease and remission aren't the only options—I am proof that lupus can be cured.

 ## You Have the Power to Heal

The healing path is uniquely yours: it has forks, crossroads, diversions, varying speeds, yield and stop signs. Yet, you must stay the course to reach your destination; it is the journey that heals. You are the decision-maker and will make the best decisions for yourself. Trust in yourself. Diversions will take you off-course—expect them—but know that you will return and continue. There are no shortcuts; be patient and steadfast in your commitment to yourself. Don't let fear divert your path. Trust yourself and your innate ability to heal. When fear emerges, take it as a sign to look inward for insight. Listen and follow your inner wisdom.

There are multiple aspects to healing: faith, trust, determination, belief, self-reliance, conviction, loss, anger, frustration, discouragement, and more. Welcome each as they visit you. They are part of the teachings of healing. If you learn from them, you move forward; if not, you will repeat the lesson until you've learned it. Be vigilant and remain anchored to your vision.

> **I have been a seeker, and I still am,**
> **but I stopped asking the books and the stars.**
> **I started listening to the teaching of my Soul.**
> **—RUMI**

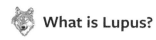 **What is Lupus?**

According to the Lupus Foundation of America website, lupus is a complex autoimmune disease that, as of 2023, remains incurable. However, significant advancements have been made since the time of my own diagnosis in the 1980s.

The prognosis for lupus has improved over the years. With close monitoring and appropriate treatment, approximately 80–90% of individuals with lupus can expect to live a normal lifespan. While it is true that there is currently no acknowledged cure for lupus, the majority of people living with the disease today can lead fulfilling lives without it being fatal.

The intensity and severity of lupus can vary among individuals. Some may experience mild cases, while others may have moderate or severe manifestations that can be more challenging to manage. Severe flare-ups do carry a higher risk and may be life-threatening.

For individuals with non-organ-threatening aspects of lupus, following their physician's instructions, adhering to prescribed medications, and being vigilant about unexpected side effects or new lupus manifestations can contribute to a normal lifespan. Hospitalization is rarely required for most individuals with lupus, especially those who maintain a healthy lifestyle.

The field of lupus research continues to yield new and unexpected findings each year. The progress made in the last decade alone, in terms of treatment and diagnosis, has surpassed that of the previous century. As such, it is prudent to strive for disease management and control, as tomorrow may bring new possibilities for a potential widespread cure.

If you're unfamiliar with lupus or only have a limited understanding of it, you're not alone. To help you gain clarity and a deeper understanding, Chapter 11 provides a more in-depth overview of lupus.

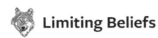 ## Limiting Beliefs

At the start of my journey, fear and self-doubt plagued me. Although I knew deep down that healing was possible, I was easily influenced and initially placed my trust in the conventional science and research model. I found myself oscillating between following my inner compass and listening to the advice of the doctors I had at the time.

In retrospect, I believe that it was these limiting beliefs and my tendency to second-guess my inner physician that kept me trapped in a state of illness. The limiting beliefs were not truly mine; they had been imposed upon me by well-meaning family, friends, and the medical community. Although their intentions were good, the fear-based and self-doubting beliefs would have kept me sick, preventing me from being here today, writing this book.

Despite the lack of belief from others, I held steadfast faith in myself. However, it was not easy to stay on course. The journey was challenging and exhausting as I continually sought to assure everyone that I knew what I was doing. My youth and deep respect for those concerned about me led me to second-guess myself frequently. I became preoccupied with worries about others' opinions when I explored nontraditional healing methods. Allowing their beliefs to sway me, I began to view my efforts as futile, potentially harmful wishful thinking, or even pseudoscience. Consequently, my healing and happiness came to a halt.

It was during this time that I realized the importance of anchoring myself in my own beliefs. However, before I could do so, I needed to gain crystal clarity on what those beliefs truly were. I had to establish firm boundaries, fully aware that this process would inevitably change many of my relationships. At a certain point, I made the decision to draw a line in the sand. Those who were willing to support me and be by my side were welcome, while those who did not share my beliefs were not. It was a lonely road to traverse. However, when I finally broke free from the opinions of others and embarked on my healing path, guided by the wisdom of my soul backed with copious research, I experienced true healing. In the words of a traditional Buddhist teaching, "When your faith becomes stronger than your fears, then your dreams can become a reality."

After my diagnosis, I made a conscious choice not to give power to the limiting words used by my doctors at the time, and I refused to embrace a label. I rejected a system that wished to label me and disregard my life by assigning an expiration date, instead of believing in me and supporting my healing journey. The medications prescribed by my doctors at the time only made me feel worse and disconnected me from my higher self.

Through deep introspection and spiritual guidance, I found the path that reshaped my life and motivated me to pen this book. Optimal wellness emerges from the dynamic balance of the mind, body, and emotions, sustained by the guidance of our souls. Change your beliefs, connect with your higher self, and heal your body. Embrace curiosity; the unknown may hold your greatest lessons. Be discerning, question, listen, learn, determine, test, and share the gift of healing with the world. Remember the mantra that guided me as well: "A diagnosis is only a name given to a set of symptoms, not a death sentence."

How to Use This Book

Healing is an ongoing and evolving experience. Once you declare your intention to heal, you will take small, meaningful steps every day to nurture that declaration. Within these pages, you will find powerful and concise techniques to add to your self-help toolkit. You will free yourself from the limitations of past narratives and discover strategies to stimulate healing in your mind, body, and emotions. Use this book as a starting point for your healing journey and a means to connect with your higher self for daily guidance and inspiration.

Remember to be gentle with yourself throughout this process; true transformation takes time. Embrace small, disciplined, and consistent steps as they promise growth and progress. If you find yourself deviating from the path, acknowledge it without judgment and consciously decide to resume your journey. Reconnect with your intentions by reading your journal pages, and then reflect on your digression, reaffirming your renewed commitment to yourself.

This book is a unique blend of memoir and self-help, offering you the story of one person's personal journey intertwined with actionable steps for your own healing. The chapters have been structured in a way that allows you to use this book as a divination tool. Simply close your eyes, open to a random section intuitively, and embrace the experience and application that unfolds. The suggestions and exercises provided are concise and written with ease of implementation in mind.

During my own healing journey, I understood the limitations of having little energy or focus. Consequently, I wrote this book with your needs in mind. I wanted it to be a valuable resource that you could easily navigate, without having to sift through a lengthy memoir. While I share parts of my healing journey to offer clarity and insight into the action exercises, the focus remains on providing you with practical information and guidance to facilitate your own self-healing.

Throughout the book, you will encounter exercises carefully crafted to create awareness, ignite inspiration, and serve as keys that unlock the answers you seek on your healing path. As you engage in these exercises, you will start to notice subtle yet consistent shifts toward healing. These may manifest as increased energy, reduced pain, a more positive attitude, greater clarity regarding your next steps, and enhanced confidence in your actions.

I recommend dedicating one to three sessions per week to work through the exercises. Over time, you will naturally gravitate toward certain exercises, feeling drawn to repeat them as they resonate deeply with you. Additionally, some exercises may initially evoke a sense of unfamiliarity or discomfort. I encourage you to embrace these moments of discomfort, as they often indicate areas where you need the most healing and growth.

By embarking on this journey with an open heart and a willingness to engage in the exercises provided, you will unlock the transformative power within yourself and discover the profound potential for healing that exists within you. Enjoy reading, and may this book serve as a guide to your healing and self-discovery.

Creating a Healing Space

Establishing a sacred space dedicated to your healing work sends a powerful message to your subconscious mind and body: you are prioritizing your healing journey and embracing self-love and self-care. This sacred space becomes a haven for your mind and body, promoting a sense of calm and supporting your healing process.

Here are some suggestions for creating your healing space:

- *Healing altar:* Set up a healing altar using items that bring you peace and comfort. It can be a simple space adorned with an altar cloth, a candle, meaningful articles from loved ones, a cherished photograph, a statue, a crystal, a plant, or any item that elicits a sense of tranquility and positive energy.

- *Ritual and atmosphere:* Begin each journaling session or healing practice in your sacred space by lighting a candle, ringing a bell, or using aromatherapy to create a sensory experience. Embrace silence for a serene ambiance, or if preferred, play soft instrumental music to aid relaxation. Remember, this space is entirely yours, so feel free to customize it to your preferences.

- *Location and ambiance:* Choose a location for your sacred space that resonates with you. It can be a small corner in your bedroom, a cozy nook in a closet, or any area where you can find serenity. Make it your favorite place to retreat to. Keep your sacred space clean, bright, and free from any distractions that may disrupt your intentional positive energy. Keep the setup simple and comfortable, allowing enough room to lie down if desired, and consider using pillows to support your back during journaling or meditation. Consider creating a beautiful hand-drawn sign to hang on the door when you're engaged in your healing work, ensuring uninterrupted privacy and focus.

- *Supporting presence:* If you feel inclined, welcome the essence of guiding energies, memories of loved ones, or any comforting presence. Invite those with whom you feel safe and supported to be with you during your introspective journey in this special space.

By intentionally creating and nurturing your sacred healing space, you are cultivating an environment that honors and supports your well-being. It becomes a sanctuary where you can connect with your inner self, embark on transformative healing practices, and find solace and rejuvenation along your journey.

Embrace the opportunity to create this sacred space as a testament to your commitment to self-care and healing. May it serve as a constant reminder of the profound healing potential that resides within you.

Your Healing Journal

I encourage you to keep a journal to document your healing journey. A three-ring notebook binder is ideal, as it allows you to add pages and organize your entries. You can personalize the cover with a title like "My Healing Journey," or choose a beautifully designed premade journal that resonates with you.

Your journal will serve as a chronological record of your progress. Revisiting past exercises and journal entries holds immense value. It allows you to reflect on how far you've come and provides motivation during challenging times.

Here's a suggested approach to journaling:

- *Date and record:* Begin each entry by dating it and capturing the experiences, emotions, triggers, and symptoms you've encountered throughout the day. Consider the mental, physical, emotional, and spiritual aspects of your well-being.

- *Healing intention:* Set a healing intention for the day. It can be a specific focus or affirmation that aligns with your healing goals and aspirations. This intention will guide your actions and mindset as you move through the day.

- *Exercise responses:* Use your journal to record your responses to the exercises provided in this book. Write down your thoughts, insights, and realizations. Capture any shifts in your perspectives, beliefs, or behaviors that occur as a result of these exercises. Your journal is a safe space to express your deepest feelings, explore ingrained beliefs, share your thoughts, and document your dreams.

- *Change and growth:* Your journal will serve as a testament to your progress. Acknowledge and celebrate the positive changes and growth you experience along your healing journey.

Recognizing these milestones will reinforce your commitment to the path of healing.

Your journal is your trusted companion and ally throughout your healing process. It allows you to observe patterns, track your transformation, and honor your innermost thoughts and experiences. Revisit your journal regularly to remind yourself of the progress you've made and to find inspiration during challenging times.

Embrace the power of journaling as a tool for self-reflection, self-expression, and self-discovery. May your journal serve as a valuable resource and witness to your profound healing journey.

The Power of Affirmations

Affirmations play a significant role in the exercises throughout this book. They serve as powerful tools for shifting your beliefs and ultimately transforming your actions.

Affirmations are conscious statements that support us in reaching our desired outcomes. By repeating affirmations throughout the day, we are making a deliberate declaration of what we intend to manifest. You can use the affirmations provided as a starting point and tailor them to align with your specific healing goals. Remember, this is your unique healing journey, and the exercises and suggestions are meant to inspire and guide you.

To effectively work with affirmations, consider the following instructions and suggestions:

- *Speak in the present:* State your affirmations as though you have already achieved the desired goal. For example, if you were given a terminal diagnosis but choose to believe in your healing, you can affirm: "I *am* healed. I *am* healthy. I *am* whole." Repeat these affirmations several times a day, allowing them to resonate within you. By speaking in the present tense, you align your thoughts and actions with the belief that you are already healed. This affirmation becomes your reality, influencing every aspect of your life.

- *Repetition and action:* Changing our beliefs requires repetition and consistent action toward the new belief. By repeating affirmations, they become embedded in our subconscious, gradually replacing undesirable beliefs. As you affirm your desired outcome, accompany it with aligned actions. Let your beliefs guide your decisions and behaviors, reinforcing the positive change you seek.

- *Personalize and empower:* Feel free to modify the affirmations provided to resonate with your unique healing journey. Tailor them to reflect your highest desired outcome and use language that speaks directly to your soul. Personalized affirmations carry immense power and create a deeper connection with your healing intentions.

By consciously choosing positivity over pessimism and aligning our thoughts and actions, we tap into our inherent ability to achieve anything. Affirmations serve as a powerful tool to rewire our beliefs, cultivate a positive mindset, and manifest the healing we desire.

Embrace affirmations as a daily practice, allowing their transformative energy to permeate your thoughts, feelings, and actions. Through consistent repetition and aligned action, you harness the power to create positive change and realize your healing potential.

Affirm your healing journey and embrace the limitless possibilities that lie ahead. You are the author of your own story, and affirmations are the ink that empowers you to script a life of wellness and wholeness.

Listening to Yourself

It is essential to listen to and honor the signs your mind, body, and spirit give you. They hold the wisdom of what is best for you. While this book is based on what worked for me, it is crucial for you to discern what resonates with your unique journey. Take from it what works for you and leave the rest, as our paths to healing will be different. Throughout the book, you will find suggestions and action steps designed to initiate healing in your mind, body, and soul. The goal is to align these aspects, because when one is out of balance, it affects the others and can create dis-ease.

If you are new to practices such as setting intentions, using affirmations to shift beliefs, embracing positivity, exploring spirituality, or engaging in energy healing, embrace the newness with an open mind and a curious spirit. As you apply the exercises, you will tap into the infinite knowledge and guidance of your soul's wisdom.

While this book offers guidance, let me stress again that it is essential to consult with your medical doctor to ensure that the techniques presented here will not cause harm or interfere with any ongoing medical treatments.

Remember, there are no shortcuts to healing, and setbacks and derailments are to be expected along the way. Have faith in the process. Embrace the moments of awkwardness and discomfort, knowing that they are often the precursors to growth, change, and healing. It is on the other side of these challenges that we often find profound transformation.

Trust yourself, trust the journey, and remain open to the possibilities that lie ahead. Your healing is a sacred unfolding, and by listening to yourself and embracing the discomfort that comes with growth, you will discover the resilience and strength that reside within you.

Navigating Discomfort in the Quest for Healing

In the intricate dance of healing, comfort zones are often tested. The journey, far from being linear, is more like a winding path with ups and downs. One of the most pressing challenges we face is deciphering the nature of our discomforts. Are they signals to retreat or signs that we're on the brink of transformation?

Determining whether a challenge in your healing journey is a standard setback or a sign that the current approach is unsuitable can be complex. Here are some pointers to help discern:

- *Duration and intensity:* Normal setbacks may be temporary and may dissipate after some time. If the issue persists or intensifies over an extended period, it could be more than a mere setback.

- *Frequency:* Experiencing the same issues repeatedly despite taking measures to address them could indicate a more significant problem with the current approach.

- *External factors:* Sometimes, external factors like stress, changes in the environment, or other life events can contribute to a setback. It's essential to consider these when evaluating the nature of the setback.

- *Your body's overall response:* If, apart from the setback, you notice other positive changes or improvements in your overall health and well-being, the setback might be a part of the healing process. However, if your overall well-being starts declining, it may be time to reconsider the approach.

- *Expert opinion:* Consulting with healthcare or wellness professionals you trust can provide clarity. They might offer insights based on their expertise and provide perspective on whether what you're experiencing is a typical part of the process or something more concerning.

- *Comparative analysis:* Using your healing journal, compare your current experience to previous times when you've encountered setbacks. Are the sensations or symptoms more severe? Are they affecting your daily life more than before?

- *Instincts and intuition:* Your body and mind have an innate wisdom that will guide you on your healing journey. If something feels off, listen to your intuition. It may be more than just a minor hiccup.

- *Adaptability:* Remember that healing isn't always linear. If, after a setback, you adapt your strategies and see improvement, it is a part of the process.

Determining whether to stay the course or change direction in your healing journey is a blend of monitoring physical and emotional responses, seeking expert guidance, and tuning into your intuition. Being patient, observant, and proactive in seeking understanding and solutions is crucial.

Problematic Potentials

On a self-healing journey, you must be aware of warning signs that might indicate you're on the wrong path. While everyone's experience is unique, some common warning signs include:

- *Worsening symptoms:* If the steps you're taking lead to a deterioration of your symptoms rather than improvement, it's a red flag.

- *Increased fatigue:* If your fatigue is worsening or becoming more intense, even with adequate rest, it might signal that the current healing approach exacerbates your condition.

- *Persistent pain:* Any new or intensified pain that persists can be a warning that the approach is not suitable for you.

- *Mental and emotional distress:* Increased anxiety, depression, or other emotional disturbances might be a sign to reconsider your approach.

- *Digestive issues:* If you're trying a new diet or supplement and you notice persistent stomach problems, bloating, or changes in bowel habits, these could be warning signs.

- *Adverse reactions:* Rashes, breathing difficulties, or other allergic reactions can indicate a particular treatment or approach is unsuitable for you.

- *Lack of progress:* If you see no progress or improvement after your expected time frame, it's worth re-evaluating your healing strategy.

- *Overdependence on a single method:* Relying too heavily on one approach without considering a holistic or comprehensive plan can signify an imbalanced healing journey.

- *Ignoring professional advice:* If you're consistently going against advice from experts you trust without seeing positive results, consider if your chosen path is the best for your situation.

If you recognize any of these signs, it's crucial to pause, reassess, and consider seeking guidance from trusted individuals. Remember, self-healing is a personal journey, and what works for one person might not work for another.

Lessons from Setbacks

While most of us yearn for an unhindered journey, setbacks often serve a greater purpose than just signaling mistakes. They spotlight aspects we may have missed, bestowing invaluable lessons.

Every experience is a teacher, and my own lessons became strikingly evident when I decided to ramp up my exercise routine. My body's immediate response? Overwhelming fatigue and pronounced inflammation. Rather than dismissing these signs, I interpreted them as my body's way of underlining the importance of hydration and caution against overexertion.

Another lesson came when I attempted to address overgrowth of a type of yeast called candida. In the process, I was blindsided by a Herxheimer reaction, an intense response to the candida die-off in my body. Similarly, after overindulging in junk foods I had abstained from for a while during a friend's party, my joints retaliated with inflammatory pain for several days.

Though these situations initially felt like setbacks, they eventually became luminous markers, highlighting the significance of maintaining a disciplined balance and closely listening to my body's communication. Disruptions, though they may catch us off-guard, can often lead us to a clearer understanding. They remind us of the need for balance, resilience, and the continuous refinement of our wellness strategies.

Here are some journaling questions to gain clarity regarding your setbacks:

- *Duration of symptoms:* How long have you experienced these symptoms compared to previous episodes? Are they short-lived, or do they linger for an extended period?

- *Frequency:* How often do you experience these symptoms now compared to before? Are they sporadic, or have they become a constant presence?

- *Triggers:* Are there any identifiable triggers that have caused these symptoms in the past and now? Has the nature or number of triggers changed?

- *Coping mechanisms:* What strategies or remedies worked in the past? Are they still effective, or do you need new methods?

- *Intensity fluctuations:* Have there been periods where the symptoms eased? If so, how does that compare to past experiences?

- *Emotional and mental impact:* Beyond the physical, how are these symptoms affecting your mental and emotional well-being compared to previous instances? Are feelings of anxiety, stress, or frustration more pronounced?

- *External influences:* Are there any external factors (such as changes in personal relationships, work stress, or environment) that might have influenced these symptoms now and in the past?

- *Support systems:* How have your support systems (such as friends, family, or professional networks) been instrumental during these times? Is their role different now than in previous episodes?

- *Interventions:* Have you tried any new treatments or interventions since the last setback? How do they compare in effectiveness?

- *Progress indicators:* Despite the setbacks, can you identify areas of improvement or progress when you compare your current situation with past experiences?

Discomfort, in all its forms, stands as a testament to healing. Instead of being an obstacle, it's an open invitation to confront, mend, and evolve. The healing journey isn't rooted in baseless optimism but in a profound trust in one's inherent strength and the comprehensive essence of healing. This unwavering faith is our navigational star, guiding us even in challenging terrains.

Choosing to Adjust or Pivot

In the healing odyssey, crossroads are inevitable: do you recalibrate your tactics or opt for a new direction? Here's guidance for such decisions:

- *Note the duration and intensity:* A fleeting discomfort might be natural, but lingering or escalating pain necessitates a reevaluation.

- *Revisit your Healing Journal:* This record is your guide. Re-examining its contents can unveil trends, aiding in informed choices.

- *Seek expert counsel:* A fresh viewpoint can shed light on overlooked nuances from someone who has triumphed on your path or from a seasoned professional.

- *Assess holistic well-being:* If an approach drains you mentally or emotionally, its long-term feasibility becomes questionable.

- *Listen to your inner voice:* Your intuition holds profound wisdom. Trust in that inner compass, and you'll find it to be a beacon of clarity in the midst of uncertainty.

- *Inspect the grand scheme:* Sometimes, the key isn't discarding an approach but refining its nuances. The choice between minor adjustments and a complete overhaul often intertwines with factual assessments, expert counsel, and personal gut feeling.

Healing is a journey tailored to the individual. What's transformative for one person might not resonate with another. It's vital to stay fluid, remain receptive, and shower yourself with kindness throughout this deeply personal expedition. Every healing voyage is an individual masterpiece, an intricate weave of diverse experiences. The necessity is to be astute, fathom discomforts, and move forward judiciously. In doing so, the hurdles and discomforts we grapple with often metamorphose into agents of significant growth and profound healing. Cherish the expedition, trust the unfolding, and let each step, however tentative, be a leap toward transformation.

Your Morning Healing Ritual

Take time in your healing space each morning to get centered and connected with your higher self, your inner physician. After you have prepared the space by lighting your candle, turning on music, or whatever else you do to create a sense of beginning:

Get comfortable in your seat.

Close your eyes, place your hands at the center of your chest (your heart center), and focus on connecting with your heartbeat. Take your time.

Take several slow deep breaths, inhaling deeply and exhaling fully. Then—silently or quietly to yourself—say, "Mind, body, soul," as if you were counting to three. Repeat for each of the following breath counts.

Begin by slowly inhaling for three counts, then holding your breath for three, slowly exhaling for three, then holding the exhale for three, and repeat this series until you feel centered and relaxed. Focus on connecting with your heart center, relaxing your mind, and letting go of any tension in your body.

Once you feel relaxed, slowly open your eyes and read your affirmation aloud, remembering to state it with conviction as if it's currently true. For example: "I *am* healthy. I *am* healed. I *am* whole." Then, upon inhaling, silently repeat the affirmation, letting the words and breath permeate your body with your belief. Hold your breath for a count of three, then upon exhalation repeat it again silently with the intention of exhaling the belief into the universe. Connect with how you feel as you decree your affirmation.

Remember to smile *and connect* with each word and your mind, body, and spirit as you repeat. Connect with your bodily sensations, sit as long as desired, and focus on *feeling* what the affirmation imparts to your mind, body, and spirit.

End each session with a blessing of gratitude.

Let's begin! Most exercises should be performed in your healing space using the steps above.

Chapter 1

THE FIRST STEPS

**Our deepest fear is not that we are inadequate.
Our deepest fear is that
we are powerful beyond measure.
It is our light, not our darkness,
that most frightens us.**
—MARIANNE WILLIAMSON

When we acknowledge and document where we are when we begin our healing journey, we become acutely aware of our own beliefs, desires, and intentions. In today's social media age, it's easy to be swayed by others' beliefs and become confused, fearful, and distracted, prompting both indecisiveness and procrastination. By taking the time to honor yourself, you're gaining clarity, discovering your highest intention for yourself, and anchoring to your decision.

Begin by retreating to your prepared healing space and journaling answers to the questions below. It's essential that you are crystal clear about *where* you are starting from and precisely what you want for yourself.

These first steps are the foundation for a successful healing journey. In addition, your answers serve as a comparison point to measure progress. Please date each entry and answer each question as best you can, even if it's just a short sentence. Some questions may remain blank, and that's okay. You can come back to them at a later time and try again. Remember to stay connected with your heart center (see the introduction for specifics) and tune in to how you *feel*—body, mind, and spirit. Note these feelings on the sidelines of the paragraph.

Start with Your "Why"

Start your paragraph with: "I am reading *Starving the Wolf* because..." then answer the following questions:

- What diagnosis are you labeled with? Describe your immediate thoughts and response to hearing this diagnosis. How did you *feel* when you received the diagnosis? Where did you *feel* this reaction in your body? What was your initial response to the diagnosis (denial, keeping it to yourself, fear, overwhelm, etc.)?

- What were the first signs that something was out of balance? How long had you been suffering, including the time before deciding to go to a doctor? Recall in detail. Describe how it progressed and what prompted you to go for testing.

- Do you know what triggered your condition? Did you experience a stressful or traumatic event prior to the onset of symptoms? How were you treating yourself? Were you in a stressful relationship?

- What is *your* current belief about the diagnosis?

- What steps have you taken to heal yourself thus far, and what were the outcomes of these actions? Please list all of them. Did you invest yourself fully in these action steps, or did your commitment fade? If so, why? Why did you change course or lose faith in your initial decision? Why didn't you stay committed?

- Describe how you are feeling today. What makes you feel better, and what makes you feel worse? How do you feel mentally, emotionally, physically, and spiritually?

- Describe your current medical protocol and how it makes you feel physically, mentally, and emotionally.

- What medications and supplements are you currently taking?

- What is your current diet? Write down everything you've put in your mouth over the past week, including not just meals but water, alcohol, gum, candy, etc.

- How is your energy level on a typical day? What depletes your energy? What energizes you?

- How is your sleep? How do you feel when you wake up each morning?

- What is your current life situation in the following areas:

    — *Work life*   — *Love life*

    — *Social life*   — *Self-care*

    — *Family life*

- Do you feel supported on your healing journey? If so, by whom?

- Is there anyone you wish supported you differently? Who is it, and how does this make you feel?

- What are your fears surrounding your diagnosis? What are your worries about your future?

- What inspired you to take charge of healing yourself?

- Compared to how you are today, how do you visualize yourself one year from now?

- What is your biggest dream or desire that would "light you up" once you achieved it?

Reading through your journal during the healing process will instill renewed hope. We tend to forget where we began, especially when we've been feeling good for a while, then briefly slip back into old habits and have previous symptoms resurface. We blame and create excuses for why we're sick again and doubt that what we're doing is working. When we're experiencing a healing crisis and read through our journal, we gain respect and appreciation for our progress and are inspired to continue forging ahead.

Become a Body Detective

Awaken your innate problem-solver. Become a detective of your own body and question everything. Leave no stone unturned; anything can affect your immune system's functionality. I've put this section here purposefully: when you ask the questions below, you'll find that your inspiration to heal yourself will be amplified. Knowing that you can explore multiple areas of your life to boost your healing power is empowering and instills hope.

By questioning everything in my life, I became acutely aware of the various possibilities that could have triggered or supported me staying sick. I was driven by my desire to live, not just with fewer symptoms but without any symptoms at all. I wasn't asking myself these questions to create guilt or blame myself; I felt empowered when I asked the hard questions and gave fully honest answers. I also realized I had more control over my healing than I previously thought. Questioning myself helped me become self-reliant in my recovery.

The following questions will help you to begin your self-investigation, self-discovery, and contemplation; you may even find yourself adding questions to the list as you go through it. Although this is an extensive inquiry list, let it serve as a starting point. If you don't have an immediate answer or knowledge of what the questions are asking, take time to explore these areas further to obtain the answers. Make sure you investigate everything possible. Be mindful that life moves on a continuum between thriving and death as you answer them. Also consider asking yourself if what you're doing is helping you to thrive, or if it is supporting illness.

- Are you drinking or eating something too often? (Take note if you often give in to cravings for sweet, salty, creamy, crunchy foods, or caffeine or alcoholic beverages.)

- Are you eating in a stressful environment?

- Are you properly digesting what you're eating? Do you feel great after you eat, or are you experiencing headaches, belching, bloating, abdominal pain, fatigue, etc.?

- Do you have constipation or diarrhea often?

- Are you vitamin- or mineral-deficient? Deficiencies have a huge impact on your overall health. Ask your doctor to run a nutritional profile, or hire a functional or naturopathic physician to assist you in obtaining these lab results.

- Are you taking supplements or herbal remedies? If so, list them, then write down why you're taking each, how long you've been taking them, and how they're affecting you.

- Are you dehydrated? Is your urine scant and dark colored, are you lightheaded, or do you have a dry mouth?

- Is your drinking and bathing water toxic? Your local Department of Health or Environmental Protection Agency office can provide you with resources and testing results.

- Are your foods nutrient dense?

- Do you over- or under-eat?

- Are you concerned with where your food comes from? Are you eating organic food?

- Do you obsess about your weight or looks?

- Which foods make you feel great? Which make you feel gastric distress? Which make you feel tired?

- Did you recently have surgery? How about dental work? Do you have amalgam fillings?

- Are you sleeping next to your cell phone as it charges?

- Are you sleeping on a heating pad?

- Did you recently purchase a new bed, carpeting, or furniture?

- Are you using toxic laundry soap or fabric softener?

- Are you sleeping or spending a lot of time on a geopathic stress line?

- Do you sleep well? If not, what's disturbing your sleep?

- Are you working in a toxic environment—chemically, emotionally, or other?

- Is mold making you sick?

- Do pets sleep in your bedroom with you?

- Are you angry or thinking negative thoughts?

- Are you breathing shallowly?

- Are you neglecting your self-care?

- Do you worry often? Are you constantly stressed out?

- Are you sad? Lonely?

- Are you always in a hurry, feeling there's not enough time?

- Have you abused your body?

- Do you disregard your needs or put others' needs first?

- Are you too aggressive or overly passive?
- Are you resentful?
- Are you self-critical?
- Were you abused—emotionally, physically, or sexually?
- Have you given up hope?
- Do you carry guilt or shame?
- Do you carry burdens from childhood?
- Are you in a toxic relationship?
- Are you a victim of your past?
- Do you sit all day?
- Do you excessively exercise?
- Do you obsess over anything?
- Do you punish yourself or self-sabotage your efforts?
- Are you a perfectionist?
- Do you believe that *others* should tend to your health?
- Do you have a virus suppressing your immune system?
- Have you taken antibiotics recently?
- Are you taking medications daily?
- Do you use insecticide?
- Are you allergic to your pet?
- Is your home dust-filled?
- Do you have a spiritual practice?
- Are you happy in your relationships?
- Are you happy at work?
- Where do you feel your best? Worst? (Relating to a specific physical space, person(s) or alone, etc.)

As you can see, this list can be exhaustive and your journal entries should leave no stone unturned. Your goal is to deeply explore your life in all of its aspects to see where you may be experiencing imbalance.

 ## Ask Yourself If You Are Ready to Heal

And now, the most important question of all: are you ready to heal? This is a profound reflective question, so take your time answering it. You may uncover why you have yet to heal.

Sometimes an illness shows up to protect us from an outcome we fear. In some way, the sickness is comforting and fulfills an underlying need. For example, if we feel lonely, undesired, disrespected, or undervalued, chronic illness might manifest as a way of fulfilling the need to feel love and belonging. It gives us something to identify with and receive attention for. A disease teaches us about ourselves and encourages spiritual growth. It demonstrates a lack of harmony somewhere in our system. Not all illness is emotionally charged, but being aware of your feelings is one of the healing keys.

Connecting with our feelings surrounding something we want to change opens us to limitless possibilities. But conversely, being unaware and closed to exploring our feelings prevents growth. Be patient and allow yourself to feel. Let your inner physician and wisdom guide your healing. You have the answers and can fulfill your desires regardless of where you are beginning. Ask yourself, "Am I *ready* to heal on every level of my being?" If you hear a resounding "I AM!" then answer the following questions:

- What has this illness prevented you from becoming, doing, believing, and enjoying?

- How does the thought of healing your body make you feel?

Excited? Nervous? Positive? Scared? Unsure? Overwhelmed? Determined? Connect with your emotions and journal without censoring.

- Why heal now? Journal why you decided to take full responsibility for healing your body. Begin sentences with "I am."

If you discover that you're not quite ready to heal, then ask yourself, "What needs to change so that I *am* ready to heal? What do I need to do to initiate this change?" Now list twenty-five reasons you desire to heal, listing all of life's joys and pleasures that you're missing out on because of this illness. Write as many sentences as necessary to complete this section, beginning each sentence with: "I am ready to heal myself because..." using reasons from the list above.

Declare *what* you are healing with specificity and as though you've already accomplished it. Describe what you healed using *your* language instead of medical terms, and state them in the past tense. Include beliefs, symptoms, emotions, traumas, etc. Don't be concerned with how; once you decree it, the how will unveil itself. Instead, focus your intention on precisely what the outcome is. Your intention is the momentum of your healing.

Write as many decrees as desired. Examples include: "I healed inflammation in my body." "I healed the exhaustion I felt in my mind and body." "I healed the thoughts and beliefs that contributed to this illness." "I healed past traumas that contributed to my weakened body." "I healed by transforming my anger into action." Continue listing everything you desire to heal, getting clearer and more specific as you list them; reiteration is welcomed.

Finally, ask, "What will my life be like when I am healed?" For this question, set aside a half-hour, close your eyes, and visualize your ideal healthy, joy-filled, successful life. Where are you? Who are you with? What are you doing? How do you feel? Take plenty of time and *see* yourself *doing* everything you desire. Deeply connect with what it *feels like* to have what you desire. Connect with the energy of your authentic life as you see it in vivid detail. Then journal the answer to the question above.

 ## Create a Vision Board

Remember that everything is possible. If you can envision it, you can create it. A vision board anchors you to the energy of your desires.

Using a 24" x 36" poster board, scissors, glue, markers, and a pile of magazines, create a vision of your desired life. Declare a date to achieve your vision and write it in the center of the poster board.

Take a picture of yourself and glue it at the top. Flip through magazines and tear and trim images and phrases representing your desired life. Then assemble and glue them on the poster board, arranging them as desired. You can group them by personal achievements, family, travel, business, etc. If you would like, add positive affirmations with markers in any blank spots.

Proudly display the board in your sacred healing space and take time daily to connect with your desires by looking at the images and recalling the steps you've taken toward the goal thus far. Then proclaim what your next step is toward achieving it, and say a prayer of gratitude for your progress. As you achieve a goal, take a marker and draw a big smiley face over the image that represents it.

REMEMBER:
A diagnosis is just a name given to a set of symptoms;
it's not a death sentence.

Find Those Who Support Your Healing Vision

Not everyone has someone to stand by their side and support them as they go through the healing journey. Friends and loved ones mean well. They believe they know what's best for us and what our path should be. Yet not all of them will be on board with you when you make choices that are different from the norm.

Surround yourself with those who support your vision of healing. This is a time to create firm boundaries. Proclaim your healing path and request that they respect your decision. Surround yourself with loving, nurturing supporters, both among your personal friends and within the medical community, and be discerning with those who challenge you, as they may unintentionally weaken your resolve.

 ## Raise Your Energy and Connect with Your Higher Self

When I refer to raising our energy or frequency, I'm referring to the energy field within and surrounding our body. This field is affected by our thoughts and the thoughts of others. We are energetic beings, souls in a body. Our body reflects our thoughts. Our thoughts are energy. We can't see the energy of thought, but we can see what thoughts manifest.

Thoughts can increase or deplete our energy. They can make us well or create illness. Others' thoughts can affect our energy as well; our energy field overlaps with others when we're near one another, and if someone else is struggling with fear or cynicism, this can affect our own energy.

Have you ever said to yourself, "I don't know why I'm feeling this way," or "I don't know why I just said that"? Or walked into a supermarket feeling energized and happy and then walked out feeling drained, irritated, exhausted, or another negative emotion? It's possible that, without even knowing it, you've experienced a negative energy exchange while standing in the checkout line. When our energy field overlaps with someone else's, we unconsciously pick up the energy of their thoughts and emotions. Likewise, ours can permeate theirs.

Sometimes this can be a good thing, especially if someone feels gloomy and another person shares some positive, loving energy. Sharing our positive energy is great; our positive thoughts maintain a healthy field of energy in and around us. Optimistic, loving, kind, compassionate thoughts combined with positive action create higher vibrational energy around the body. Conversely, if we're feeling or subjecting this field to aggressive, pessimistic, angry, unkind, impatient thoughts and actions daily, our minds and body suffer. Remember that like attracts like: the more positive energy your thoughts and actions create, the greater the healing potential.

As a contrast, let's take the energies of joy and despair. The energy of "joy" is a high vibrational, expansive energy. When the body experiences joy, it responds with a high level of energy, and we radiate joy. Others can feel our happiness across a room. When we're joy-filled, we feel energized and excited; our heart is happily pumping, our mind is sharp, our smile infectious. Others are intrigued by our energy.

In contrast, we sense the energy of "despair" as low vibrational, contracted energy. Others may feel this despondency as depressed, draining energy and aren't drawn to us. Low vibrational energy supports sickness in the body.

Our thoughts create our energy and environment; our actions bring life to our thoughts. So be mindful of what you are thinking. Maintaining a healthy energetic balance is vital. If our energy is deficient, we get sick and eventually die, while excessive or prolonged stress can irritate, overwhelm, and inflame the body.

When I refer to your "higher self," I'm talking about that quiet part of you that seems deeply connected and insightful. People tap into this awareness in moments of deep focus, relaxation, or even when daydreaming. Have you ever driven and realized that you don't remember the specifics of the drive, yet you've arrived safely? That's a glimpse of this inner connection in action. It's an intuitive, almost automatic side of us. Some liken it to a deep intuition or a subconscious guide. It's that boundless silent center of your being. As you close this chapter, take a moment to appreciate the journey you've taken within. You've delved deep into your own world, uncovering the beliefs, attitudes, habits, and choices that shape your reality. Remember, the power to heal lies within you. Embrace the wisdom of your inner physician, and allow it to guide you on your path to wholeness.

Chapter 2

THE BELIEF OF HEALING

**Healing may not be so much about getting better,
as about letting go of everything that isn't you—
all of the expectations, all of the beliefs—
and becoming who you are.**
—RACHEL NAOMI REMEN

Five to seven years. Five to seven years! That's how long the doctor said I had to live after I was diagnosed with systemic and discoid lupus. But I refused to accept that prognosis. I was determined to rewrite my story, fueled by hope and grit. In the bold spirit of my younger years, I chose the road less taken and embraced an alternative path. Some raised eyebrows, but their doubts were like whispers against my roaring determination. I knew that healing would be a journey, not a destination. There would be ups and downs along the way. But I was determined not to give up. I believed I would heal myself.

I'm living proof that it's possible to overcome adversity and thrive. I'm grateful for every day, and I want my story to inspire you to begin your healing journey.

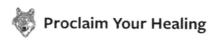 Proclaim Your Healing

> **Feeling the reality of the state sought,
> and living and acting on that conviction,
> is the way of all seeming miracles.
> All changes of expression are brought about
> through a change of feeling.**
> **—NEVILLE GODDARD**

The foundation of my healing was believing I would cure myself.

Everyone has a unique inner resilience that can play a role in their healing journey. Adopting new beliefs and a wellness mindset, and taking active steps towards better health, can have a positive impact on our well-being. However, it is important to remember that everyone's response to these things is different, and this approach alone is not a guaranteed solution for everyone. Nevertheless, when we are deeply committed to a goal, it is inspiring to see how often the outcome can exceed our initial expectations.

To begin to embody a new belief, proclaim it and then repeat that proclamation until the idea becomes you. You are not lying to yourself; you are taking control of your thoughts and reprogramming undesirable, misguided beliefs.

Sometimes we decide to change a belief, and it quickly becomes our upgraded belief; other times, it takes time. Therefore, practice conviction, patience, and repetition. Stay focused on that which you desire, not your current reality.

This exercise intends to move blocked energy and infuse your mind and body with the message that you are healed. As I mentioned in the introduction, take my experiences and make them your own. Create your own healing statements.

The body is a manifestation of energy. We are unwell when our beliefs and actions aren't in alignment with our soul's desires, creating blockage or energy stagnation. This exercise helps move blocked or stagnant energy while decreeing our healing.

 Action: Retreat to your healing space. If you didn't read the introduction, please take a moment to do so now, so that you understand your sacred healing space. Then, play some calming music and visualize the release of energy and dissolution that causes illness. Close your eyes and rest one hand on your heart center, connecting with your heartbeat, and the other on your belly, feeling the rise and fall of your abdomen with each breath you take.

Slowly scan your body from your feet to your scalp and note any areas of tension, pain, inflammation, or tightness; we'll call these energetic blocks. Then, take a moment to focus on each of them and note their size, shape, depth, color, and temperature.

Now envision a beam of radiant yellow light from the heavens permeating your entire body with warm, healing energy. See and feel it infusing your whole being. Feel its warmth expanding and begin to focus it into areas of pain or tightness, directing your breath along with the light to release the collection of blocked energy. Take slow deep breaths and slowly exhale them as you envision the accumulation of energy dispersing into little evanescent bubbles that evaporate into the universe.

Continue inhaling and exhaling slowly as you visualize and feel each energetic block dissolving, then immerse yourself in this new feeling. To end the session, silently repeat the following (or your healing statement) for as long as you desire: "I am healed, I am healthy, I am whole."

With each inhale, envision every cell of your being infused with this belief—and while exhaling, smile and say, "I am healed, I am healed, I am healed!" Then open your eyes and journal about your experience. I practiced this a minimum of twice daily, morning and evening.

Your belief that you will heal yourself fuels healing. I found it best to decree that I was healed first because it's what I wanted as my truth. I intuitively knew that my body would follow my direction once I believed and felt it.

Stay connected with your convictions and believe in yourself. Inner strength and confidence can fuel your healing. Let your sense of self be the driving force behind your recovery.

Affirmations: I AM healed, I AM healthy, I AM whole. I AM healed, I AM healed, I AM healed! If doubts arise, honor them, consciously bring yourself back into the healing energy, and repeat your affirmations—then journal about your feelings surrounding your doubts. If you haven't done visualization exercises before, this may feel awkward initially. Please trust the process. There are no limits to what you can imagine or manifest. If you can't visualize, then focus on thoughts of your desired outcome and how those thoughts make you feel. Concentrate on your breathwork and bodily sensations as you bring each desired belief or affirmation to mind.

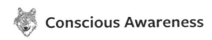 ## Conscious Awareness

Believe you can and you're halfway there.
—THEODORE ROOSEVELT

Conscious awareness is a second-by-second practice. Our thoughts and beliefs create our reality. What we believe and tell ourselves, we attract and manifest. Therefore, the foundation for optimal health is positive health-promoting thoughts.

What have you been telling yourself about yourself?

We are creators, and through our thoughts and actions, we bring things to life, either positive or negative. Take your time and reflect on each of the following questions. Check in with yourself.

- What do you think about all day long?
- What do you say to yourself when you look in the mirror?
- What are your first thoughts each morning?
- Are the majority of your thoughts optimistic and uplifting or pessimistic and cynical?

At every moment, the choice is yours. What do you choose? Be aware of what you are thinking into being. We live a happier, healthier, more vibrant life when we think positively. Our energy reflects our way of thinking. For example, when we wake each day, we may feel well-rested or groggy. Yet, regardless of how we feel, we can jump out of bed with enthusiasm to greet the new day, or grumble and pull the covers back over our heads. Whichever we decide sets the tone for the day.

When we're harsh, judgmental, and pessimistic, we deplete life force energy and attract more negativity. Like attracts like. We attract that which we think. If we think we're sick, we're fat, the world is terrible, and that is all we see—then that is what exists for us. Likewise, we thrive when we believe we are healthy and take action toward that belief by living a healthy lifestyle, seeking the best for ourselves, and loving ourselves. We begin to see life and the world in a whole new way.

Believe in miracles. Choose positivity 24/7. Change your thoughts and actions, and you change your life.

 Action: Be mindful of every word. If you're cynical and judgmental, and unkind thoughts arise, catch yourself and state, "I withdraw that statement," or "Cancel that." Then reframe and restate it into a statement aligned with your highest self. For example, if you catch yourself saying, "I'll never be able to do that," then quickly state, "I withdraw that statement," and restate, "I create my desired reality now." This practice takes conscious awareness and diligence; it is a powerful life-changing tip. Commit to it, and watch your life change significantly. It might be challenging, especially when you're chronically ill, but know that perseverance pays a colossal reward that only you can give yourself.

♡ *Affirmations:* I consciously create my life by thinking and speaking my highest choice. I take positive action steps each day toward my desired goals. As a result, my life is transforming for my highest and greatest good.

For more on conscious awareness, I recommended reading *Conscious Language: The Logos of Now* by Robert Tennyson Stevens.

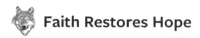 ## Faith Restores Hope

**Faith consists in believing when it is
beyond the power of reason to believe.**
—VOLTAIRE

Staying anchored to your aspirations can be challenging when grappling with chronic illness. If you sense a disconnect from your inner strength, this might be an opportune moment to reconnect and draw inspiration from those desires.

My journey through near-death experiences, illness, and healing made me deeply aware of the importance of nurturing faith in myself. Through self-reflection and meditation, I sharpened my sense of intuition and discovered pathways to healing. I realized that my inner strength and faith in myself supported recovery.

When we nurture faith in ourselves, we tap into a powerful source of resilience and hope. We become more open to the possibility of healing and are more likely to persevere in the face of challenges.

Taking time for introspection and deliberate thought can be valuable in understanding one's feelings and determining the best path forward.

 Action: Nurture your faith with the following steps.

- *Reflect on your experiences.* Take some time each day to reflect on your progress and accomplishments. This can help you to see how far you've come and to cultivate gratitude for the small moments of joy and relief.

- *Reframe challenges as opportunities for growth.* When you face challenges, view them as opportunities to learn and grow. Journal your answers to the following: What can I learn from this experience? How can I use it to become stronger and more resilient?

- *Use positive self-talk.* Affirm your strengths and resilience. Tell yourself that you are capable of overcoming anything that comes your way. State, "I am nurturing my healing, and my determination to persevere is unwavering." In your journal, write a list of your strengths. When you believe in yourself, you are more likely to persevere and achieve your healing goals.

- *Be kind to yourself and others.* Helping others is a great way to boost your own mood and sense of purpose. It can also help you to connect with others and feel more supported in your own healing journey.

- *Be patient and trust the process.* Healing takes time and effort. Don't get discouraged if you don't see results immediately. Just keep moving forward and celebrate your progress along the way.

Affirmations: Faith is my anchor. I trust the process of healing. I take care of my physical and emotional health to support my healing journey. I celebrate my successes, big and small, on the path to recovery. As a result, I am empowered to navigate the challenges and emerge stronger, embracing the joy of a healthy and fulfilling life.

Chapter 3

TAKING MINDFUL ACTION

**Love one another and help others to rise to
the higher levels, simply by pouring out love.
Love is infectious and the greatest healing energy.**
—SAI BABA

It's okay to be different and to follow your soul's guidance. Even when the naysayers don't believe in you, do it your way. It's your body.

 ## Welcome Your Loving Supporters

With an open heart, welcome all of your faithful, loving supporters. Ask them for help, guidance, and prayer.

When I was healing, most of my loved ones doubted my decision and the choices I made to heal myself. They believed that medicine was the only path to managing this disease. Their lack of support added more stress and distraction to my life. I made a conscious decision that I would discover how to heal myself, and I knew that having people in my life who challenged my choices wouldn't support my healing. I believed in myself and needed them to believe in me too. If they weren't going to be supportive, it was best we kept our distance or went our separate ways. Healing from an autoimmune disease was unheard of back in the 1980s, so I understood their concern; yet it was my path.

Surround yourself with loving, optimistic, inspiring, loyal supporters, ones who pray for your healing, believe in you, and check in on you to see how they can help. A team is great, but it only takes one loving supporter to brighten your day. Love, support, and faith encourage healing.

> **When you contact the Higher Self, the source of power within, you tap into a reservoir of infinite power.**
> **—DEEPAK CHOPRA**

 ## Self-Love

When we lack self-love, we are out of alignment with our divine self. When we are not standing in authenticity, this imbalance can manifest as an illness, relationship stress, indecisiveness, isolation, anger, depression, addiction, etc.

Love is the universal healer, and begins with a deep love of self. As we nurture ourselves with love, our immune systems strengthen, positivity and energy expand, our relationships deepen, and confidence soars. Within ourselves lies a wellspring of true, everlasting love. Self-love is the beginning of the healing journey.

Self-love is:

- essential to healing
- honoring your feelings

- forgiving yourself
- maintaining boundaries
- accepting yourself
- being kind to yourself
- welcoming change in your life
- making time each day to connect within
- asking for what you need from others
- speaking your mind
- saying "no" when desired
- being honest with yourself and others

Self-love is not:

- putting others' needs before your own
- believing that you're not enough
- neglecting your health
- judging and criticizing yourself
- carrying guilt
- sacrificing something to keep the peace
- committing to something you don't want to do
- making excuses for your actions
- feeling guilty that you desire time for yourself

The love you yearn for is within you.

Action: Consider these exercises to deepen your self-love.

- Look in a mirror and connect with your eyes. State the following or create your own statement: "I honor, respect, and love all of you. My heart is filled with love and compassion for you. Thank you for staying strong and carrying me throughout life. I promise to love and nurture you always, to treat you with kindness and respect and feed you with love-filled words and healing food."

- Stand in front of the mirror with a recording device for ten minutes. Look at yourself very slowly with admiration; start at your feet and end gazing into your eyes. Give gratitude and speak aloud about the qualities and traits you love about yourself. Take time to admire and honor God's magnificence. Mention the qualities and strengths you admire and respect in yourself. Speak as though you are speaking to a child you love dearly.

  Begin the recorder and start at your feet; give them gratitude and love for their dedication and hard work carrying you daily, etc. Slowly continue upward, showing appreciation and love to each body part. Mention specific memories you have (examples: how grateful you are for the strength in your legs and your immense gratitude for the leg that healed so quickly from the boating accident, etc.), and end by gazing into your eyes. Finish with loving appreciation for your strengths and traits (examples: what a great mother and friend you are, how committed you are to work, how great you are at self-care, how kind you are to others, etc.). Repeat this exercise weekly. Listen to the recording you made throughout the week for reinforcement.

Alternatively, sit quietly and journal, listing everything you love about yourself. Start each sentence with, "I am..." Examples: I am reliable, I am a good friend, I am dedicated, I am fun, I am intelligent, I am committed, etc. When finished, read it into a recording device and listen throughout the day for reinforcement. Practice daily and watch your self-love and self-esteem soar.

- Sit quietly and ask yourself: When did I stop loving myself? Where am I lacking in self-love? What has my inner critic been telling me? Whose voice is this (relative, boss, spouse, etc.)? How can I cultivate more compassion toward myself? Write a list of the ways you can explore self-love and self-compassion. Act on this list and revisit it weekly, adding to it as you recognize new ways to respect and honor yourself.

Relax and let go of preconceived beliefs when you do these exercises. Invite your higher self to guide and speak through you; the kind, nonjudgmental, loving side of you has much to teach you. Tapping into your authentic self may take some practice. However, being patient with yourself is an act of self-love.

Affirmations: I deeply love and care for myself. I choose to love and trust myself above all else. When I love "me," my body responds by healing. I am enough. I am perfect. I love me!

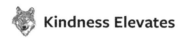 ## Kindness Elevates

**Kind words can be short and easy to speak,
but their echoes are truly endless.
—MOTHER TERESA**

Kindness eases distress and empowers us to heal. It simultaneously uplifts and energizes us. Kindness is subtle, genuine, and powerful. It bathes our lives in joy. It lowers blood pressure, reduces anxiety, and increases the capacity of our immune function to fight disease. Kindness brings us peace and revitalizes us, leading to speedier healing; it displaces heaviness and eases our suffering.

Surround yourself with kindness, and watch your healing accelerate. Smile at a stranger. Hold a door for someone without expecting anything in return. Do it because you desire to. Every morning when you open your eyes, choose kindness, and create a flow of positive change.

 Action: Perform an expanding kindness meditation in your healing space. A kindness meditation practice cultivates a deep sense of compassion and connection, bridging the gaps between ourselves and others. To do so:

- Sit or lie down in your sacred space.

- Close your eyes. Take three slow, deep breaths, letting go of external distractions and grounding yourself in the present moment. Return to your natural breath.

- Place your left hand at the center of your chest, your heart center, then place your right hand on top. Feel the gentle beating of your heart.

- With each breath, connect with the rise and fall of your chest, bringing your full attention to yourself.

- Visualize yourself as you are right now. Think of a moment when you felt peaceful. Silently say to yourself, "May I be safe. May I be content. May I be healthy. May I live with ease."

- Then bring to mind someone you deeply care about—a family member, close friend, or loved one. Visualize them smiling, and with a smile say to them, "May you be safe. May you be content. May you be healthy. May you live with ease."

- Next, think of someone you see regularly but don't know very well—perhaps a neighbor, mail carrier, or a cashier at the grocery store. Visualize them smiling, and with a smile say to them, "May you be safe. May you be content. May you be healthy. May you live with ease."

- Next, think of someone with whom you've had differences. Understand that they, too, have their struggles, fears, and hopes, just as you do. Visualize them smiling at you and with a warm smile say, "May you be safe. May you be content. May you be healthy. May you live with ease."

- Now visualize your community, then your city, your country, and finally, the entire world. Next, picture a luminous rainbow emerging from your heart, covering the sky, and wrapping around the world, brightening the spirits of everyone. Smile and silently say, "May all beings be safe. May all beings be content. May all beings be healthy. May all beings live with ease."

- Pause here, soaking in the unity of a compassionate world. When you're ready, bring your attention back to your body. Feel the weight of your body and the support beneath you. Gently move your fingers and toes. Take a couple of deep breaths, and slowly open your eyes. Take a moment to write down your thoughts, reflecting on your experience and considering ways to infuse more love and kindness into every day.

People will forget what you said, people will forget what you did, but people will never forget how you made them feel.
—MAYA ANGELOU

In your journal, write about what kindness means to you, and recall someone whom you admire for their kindness. Then, list the actions of kindness you admire in them.

Do random acts of kindness. Examples: hold a door for someone and smile; offer to carry someone's groceries; tell someone what you admire about them; hug someone; smile at strangers as you look into their eyes; send someone a cheerful card; offer to help a neighbor; volunteer at a pet rescue; feed the wild animals; brush and talk with your pet, etc.

Affirmations: I am a kind, loving, compassionate person. Kindness is the only way of life for me. Kindness fills my heart and fuels my soul.

Be kind to people who aren't.
They're the ones who need it the most.
— ZIG ZIGLAR

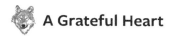 ## A Grateful Heart

**Gratitude turns what we have into enough,
and more. It turns denial into acceptance,
chaos into order, confusion into clarity...
it makes sense of our past, brings peace for today,
and creates a vision for tomorrow.**
—MELODY BEATTIE

A genuine gratitude practice improves every area of our lives. Consciously living with thankfulness each day opens us to feeling and giving more love and compassion to ourselves and others. Love heals. When we acknowledge all that we have to be grateful for, the feeling of gratefulness dilutes and overshadows the worries and unpleasantries we experience each day.

 Action: Journal each evening, listing everything you have an appreciation for that day. Be sure to list all the positive changes your body is exhibiting as it responds to the self-love and nurturing you've been giving it, including the subtle ones. Examples: you have more energy, inflammation isn't as intense as it was, you're grateful for the compassion of your loved ones, you're thankful that the sun was shining, you're grateful that you have clean water to drink, your faith, food on the table, a roof over your head, etc. This simple act of gratitude creates joy in our hearts, trickling into every part of our lives.

Next, write down how you are going to feel when you wake up the next morning. Decreeing through positive intention the evening before sets up the next day to be exactly or better than we decide it to be.

When we focus on our gratitude, the tide of disappointment goes out and the tide of love rushes in.

—KIRSTIN ARMSTRONG

Affirmations: I am filled with gratitude for the gift of life and all its blessings. I am grateful for my body's strength and resilience. I am grateful for each improvement I experience in my physical health. I am grateful for the subtle changes my body is making toward healing. My heart overflows with gratitude for the wisdom gleaned from life's journey.

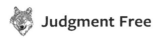

Judgment Free

**Judging is preventing us from understanding a new truth.
Free yourself from the rules of old judgments
and create the space for new understanding.**

—STEVE MARABOLI

Be curious, not judgmental.

—WALT WHITMAN

You're draining your life force energy when you cast judgment on another. When you judge others, you're avoiding acknowledging your own insecurities and where you need to change. Criticizing another disempowers you. You're robbing yourself of joy.

Being consciously aware and connected to self is a devoted practice. Questioning yourself with the intention of self-improvement is conscious awareness. When you make a conscious decision to change something about yourself that isn't in alignment with your higher self, you're supporting your spiritual growth.

**Every time I judge someone else,
I reveal an unhealed part of myself.**

—ANONYMOUS

Action: Next time you catch yourself judging some-one, close your eyes and take slow, deep breaths. Ask yourself these questions, allowing enough time in between each to hear the answers: "Why am I criticizing this person? Where might I be feeling insecure? Where can I improve myself?" and wait for an answer. Alternatively, you can ask the questions and write the answers in a journal. Remain open; it is in time of judgment that we learn the greatest gift of ourselves.

 Affirmations: I love and accept myself. I am actively releasing judgment of myself and others. I choose joy.

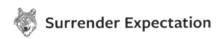 ## Surrender Expectation

**The art of surrender isn't defeat,
giving up, or powerlessness.
To surrender is choosing acceptance over resistance,
appreciation over expectations,
and flexibility over foolishness.**
—DR. FRIEDEMANN SCHAUB

Disappointment creates a cascade of toxic, obsessive thoughts that poison your body and drain your energy. Disappointment results from false expectation, which arises from deceptive beliefs, programming, fear, or insecurity. Expectation effortlessly fades when you practice surrender, faith, nonjudgment, gratitude, and forgiveness.

Perfection is an example of false expectation. Anyone can change their mind, make a mistake, break a commitment, speak out of line, forget, or tell a white lie. The illusion of perfection places great stress on you and your relationships.

You cannot predict or control the actions of another, but you can choose compassion, acceptance, and forgiveness. When we let go of preconceptions and expectations about ourselves and others, we open our minds to a broader perspective and welcome unforeseen possibilities.

**When you stop expecting people to be perfect,
you can like them for who they are.**
—DONALD MILLER

> **Expectations were like fine pottery.**
> **The harder you held them,**
> **the more likely they were to crack.**
> **—BRANDON SANDERSON**

 Action: Connect with your heart center. Finding a comfortable spot to sit, close your eyes and place your right hand on your heart center (the center of your chest), then place your left hand on top of your right hand and state the following affirmations: *I am in control of my thoughts and actions. I embrace the path that unfolds before me. I understand and accept that no one is perfect, including myself. I let go of unrealistic expectations and focus on positive personal growth. I choose acceptance, love, and compassion.*

Surrender is the ultimate sign of strength and the foundation for a spiritual life. Surrendering affirms that we are no longer willing to live in pain. It expresses a deep desire to transcend our struggles and transform our negative emotions. It commands a life beyond our egos, beyond that part of ourselves that is continually reminding us that we are separate, different, and alone. Surrendering allows us to return to our true nature and move effortlessly through the cosmic dance called life. It's a powerful statement that proclaims the perfect order of the universe.

When you surrender your will, you are saying, "Even though things are not exactly how I'd like them to be, I will face my reality. I will look it directly in the eye and allow it to be here." Surrender and serenity are synonymous; you can't experience one without the other. So if it's serenity you're searching for, it's close by. All you have to do is resign as General Manager of the Universe. Choose to trust that there is a greater plan for you and that if you surrender, it will be unfolded in time.

> **Surrender is a gift that you can give yourself.**
> **It's an act of faith. It's saying that even though**
> **I can't see where this river is flowing,**
> **I trust it will take me in the right direction.**
> **—DEBBIE FORD**

Affirmations: I release my need to control the outcome and surrender to the flow of life. I let go of all expectations and open myself to new possibilities. I am free from the burden of expectation and at peace with myself and the world around me.

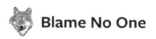 **Blame No One**

But let every man prove his own work, and then shall he have rejoicing in himself alone, and not in another. For every man shall bear his own burden.
GALATIANS 6:4–5 [KJV]

When you blame, you give your power away and convey a victim mentality. Victimhood keeps you stuck in a cyclic mode of thinking. Accepting responsibility shifts you toward a positive solution and a happier life. In addition, owning your fault frees you from the false belief that others control the outcome of your life. Commit to the decision to change old beliefs that keep you stuck.

 Action: To free yourself from the victim mentality, answer the following questions each time you find yourself blaming another for how you feel, how you think, or who you've become:

- What is the benefit of me blaming ____ for ____ ?
- How does blaming another keep me stuck in a victim mentality?
- How does remaining a victim affect my life?
- Why do I want to accept responsibility for all my actions?
- What is the benefit of changing my current belief?
- What steps can I take to change my beliefs surrounding this (event, person, situation, etc.)?

- What is the first step I am taking toward changing my belief? What are future steps I am taking toward changing my belief?

Take action on the steps indicated and journal the experiences.

Affirmations: I am accountable for all my actions. I create my happiness. I create my healthy body. I am happy with my life. I welcome positive change. I welcome personal growth.

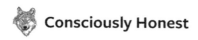 **Consciously Honest**

Honesty is the first chapter in the book of wisdom.
—THOMAS JEFFERSON

Dishonesty affects your health. Are you being honest with yourself? With others? If there were an honesty bank, how wealthy would your account be? An accumulation of deceit is toxic to the body, whether it's lying to ourselves or another.

Honesty is the foundation for living a flourishing authentic life. Speaking your truth using thoughtful language is an act of kindness. It raises your vibration and empowers you. In contrast, telling white lies, avoiding, exaggerating, and making excuses depletes energy, negatively affecting your emotions and health.

An accumulation of deceit manifests within us as uneasiness—a feeling of discontent, sadness, disconnectedness, and eventually illness. This can be seen when you find yourself saying things like "I just don't feel right," or "I can't put my finger on it."

Honesty is not blurting out your feelings when angry and hurting someone with your words. Being honest takes conscious thought, self-love, and compassion. It requires deep introspection to ask oneself: "What represents my ultimate and authentic truth?"

Sometimes the truth takes time to discern and compassionately verbalize. Mindfully take your time.

The practice of truthfulness sheds light on areas of life we're avoiding or where we are hiding. For example, perhaps you're not attending an event because you've gained some weight and your self-esteem is subdued.

The practice of speaking the truth can prompt you to act, in this case on self-care. It brings an awareness of where we're uncomfortable.

Lying keeps you stuck; truthfulness sets you free. There's deep healing in this practice.

 Action: Cultivate a daily practice of being completely honest. Begin by reflecting upon past situations where you chose to be dishonest. Just noting your actions, not judging them, journal your answers to the following:

- How did I feel in that situation?

- What prompted me to lie?

- What was I protecting when I chose to be dishonest?

- How did I feel (mentally and physically) when I lied to this person? How did I feel after I lied?

- How did I feel being in that person's presence following the lie? Did I feel guilt, fear, shame, nothing, or remorseful?

- Was I angry and disappointed in myself for lying? Where did I feel "off," uncomfortable, or have pain or tension in my body?

- How was my health affected by my dishonest actions? Did I experience insomnia, body aches, a cold, or flu symptoms shortly after that?

- What could I have said or done instead to be authentic and remain true to myself and respectful of this person?

Remember, this exercise is for your awareness and to assist your healing. Be fully honest with your answers. Your answers bring breadth and depth into the self-discovery and awareness of your actions to explore why you behave the way you do.

Accept yourself where you are and strive to be lovingly honest each day. Be gentle with yourself; it may take time to change.

Dishonesty can stem from childhood trauma where we believed that lying would protect us from pain, such as pain from disappointment, rejection, punishment, disapproval, etc.

Lying is a coping mechanism that can be changed with practice. When we consciously choose honesty, we empower ourselves, build confidence and higher self-esteem, and are trusted, respected, and energetically vibrant.

Sometimes dishonesty is a kneejerk reaction to a trigger, such as when someone brings up a past traumatic memory that we buried deep within the tissues of our body years ago, one we thought we had moved beyond but didn't. So, we avoid, deny, or blatantly lie about it. These responses affect our physical and emotional bodies. We believe that lying, avoiding, and denying protects our wounds and keeps them safe; however, keeping them repressed keeps us stuck, and it makes us sick.

Emotional toxins are stored in our cells and manifest as mental or physical illnesses. To begin to heal, acknowledge that you've been traumatized, do forgiveness work, and set yourself free. (See the "Forgiving" exercise, coming later in the book.)

Today and every day you have a choice; make it your highest. When you catch yourself about to stretch the truth—and you will—try slowing down, taking a long, slow, deep breath, and thinking before you give your answer, especially when you sense that your immediate reaction isn't genuine.

When you catch yourself in a moment where your first impulse is to be dishonest, you can simply say, "I'd like to think about this before I answer you," or "That's going to take some thought." Then, reflect deeply on your innermost feelings and motivations, and ask why you were about to be dishonest. Is it an insecurity, a false belief, or a past trauma? Take time to explore, gain clarity, and connect with the emotions and memories.

Journal on the experience.

When you catch yourself erring toward dishonesty, close your eyes and sit with the feeling, connect with your body, and note where you feel tension, constriction, or other sensations in your body. These sensations are blocked energy, which is where illness begins to manifest.

Always choose honesty; it will set you free. Take time to think about what you want to say to be honest and compassionate.

Affirmations: I respect myself and choose honesty every time. I am an honest, reliable, kind, and trustworthy person. Honesty sets me free. Honesty creates peace. I value honesty.

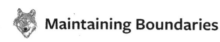

Maintaining Boundaries

To be yourself in a world that is constantly trying to make you something else is the greatest accomplishment.
—RALPH WALDO EMERSON

Knowing what your boundaries are requires you to be in touch with your feelings. When you feel anger, resentment, or discomfort in a situation, you may not be maintaining your boundaries. Ask yourself: What is it that's creating this feeling? Why am I feeling disrespected? Why am I feeling resentment toward this person? What is it that I need to say or do? What belief regarding this situation needs to change? Where am I dishonoring myself?

Action: Take time to journal about past experiences where you felt uncomfortable, passive, resentful, or frustrated with yourself for not speaking up. Recall the situation and what it was that you wanted to say, but didn't. Now, write down why you didn't express yourself. What would your highest desired outcome have been if you had asserted yourself? Write a sample of how the conversation would have gone.

Remember that you are entitled to express your desires. Expressing yourself does not make you a confrontational person. You deserve to be heard and respected. Honor yourself, and speak your truth with kindness. Practice using words to articulate how you felt and what you could say in a way that would be comfortable for you. What beliefs are you holding on to that keep you from maintaining your boundaries?

- What are your beliefs about "respect?"
- What are your beliefs about speaking to the opposite sex?
- What are your beliefs about speaking to your superiors or employers?
- What are your beliefs about speaking to elders?
- What are your beliefs about being self-confident?
- What are your beliefs about pleasing other people?
- What are your beliefs or fears surrounding speaking your mind?
- How true or false are these beliefs?

Think of someone you know and respect—someone who commands respect and maintains their boundaries. Observe them, learn from them, and emulate them. Our greatest teachers are those we admire.

Begin by practicing asserting yourself in public situations where you don't know the other person. Instead of being accommodating, express what you want. Example: You're in a restaurant having a cup of coffee and want another cup. The waitress is busy and you're hesitant to ask. When you do, she mentions that she'll have to make another pot. Instead of saying "Don't worry about it, I don't need it anyway," put your needs first and just say, "Thank you."

Another example: You're standing in line at the supermarket checkout during your lunch break. A woman with a cart filled with groceries states she's running late to an appointment and asks if she can jump in front of you. Your nature is to say, "Of course," even though you know that you've got to get back to work. Permitting her to go ahead of you reduces your lunch break and puts you under pressure. Practice being assertive and say, "I'd love to, but I can't this time." You have nothing to be sorry for, so don't apologize.

Being a doormat weakens the immune system. Don't feel guilty—value and honor yourself! Putting your needs first is self-care, not narcissism.

Depending on your upbringing or other factors, you may find it uncomfortable to assert yourself. And when you first start voicing your needs, anticipate that those in your immediate circle may feel uncomfortable. Speak your truth in love. Welcome change. Avoidance will keep you stuck, and it doesn't keep the peace. It makes you sick. Stay true to yourself. Be vulnerable; your health depends on it. Resentment creates bitterness and manifests as illness. Commit to yourself and take action. Be patient and consistent; maintaining your boundaries takes practice and perseverance.

Affirmations: I am worthy of respect and deserve to have my boundaries honored. I am comfortable saying "no" to protect my well-being. I can communicate my boundaries clearly, kindly, and assertively. I am strong enough to handle any challenges that arise from setting boundaries. Respecting my boundaries protects my energy and well-being. I am committed to maintaining healthy and respectful boundaries in all areas of my life.

Value Discomfort

Expect to be uncomfortable. Welcome the uneasiness. Healing will push you out of your comfort zone and into the uncertain. On the other side of the discomfort is expansive freedom. Trust yourself and explore the unknown. Become a courageous pioneer! Take the emotional filters off and see an abundance of opportunity. Discomfort is a catalyst for growth. Growth is a catalyst for healing. Avoidance and denial prolong pain and suffering.

Feel the pain—be it physical, situational, emotional, or spiritual—and welcome its lesson. Pain pushes us out of our comfort zone and nurtures self-reliance, self-trust, and self-liberation, leading us toward healing.

 Action: Answer the following questions in your journal:

- What am I afraid of?
- What belief prevents me from accepting change in my life?
- What am I missing out on because of this belief?
- How does having this limiting belief make me feel?
- What am I avoiding due to of my fear of discomfort?
- What are the benefits of embracing discomfort?

 Affirmations: There is great value in discomfort. I welcome change. Change is growth. Change is healthy. I embrace healthy change in my life.

> **What torments of pain have you endured
> that haven't as yet arrived? And may never!**
> **—RALPH WALDO EMERSON**

 ## Trust with All Your Heart

> **Trust yourself. Create the kind of self
> that you will be happy to live with all your life.
> Make the most of yourself by fanning
> the tiny, inner sparks of possibility
> into flames of achievement.**
> **—GOLDA MEIR**

Once you make the decision to heal your body, commit to trusting that you will. Your obedient body is relying on you to direct its healing. Vacillating on your decision or beliefs only prolongs the healing you desire.

When you willfully commit to surrender and fully trust in yourself and your body's ability to heal, your body responds enthusiastically. The body calms, feels safe, loved, and nurtured, and knows it can trust you.

When our thoughts are inconsistent with our mission, we send mixed signals to the body, and healing will halt. Your body reflects your self-talk, thoughts, and beliefs. What beliefs do you want your body to respond to? Fill your mind with thoughts that support your highest desires.

Trust in the journey, yourself, and the process. Healing takes time. There will be phases of relapse, exhaustion, pain, suffering, disappointment, and disillusionment. This is part of the healing process. Your resolve *will* be tested. Prepare for derailments by remaining firm in your faith and commitment to yourself. Anchor to your truth.

 Action: Trust your decisions. When you listen deeply to your innermost feelings and seek their guidance, you're being led by your truest self. (Refer to exercise in Chapter 5 under "Whispers of Your Soul.") Be deliberate about scheduling time for healing introspection each day. Prepare a question or two to ask your innermost self, or ask for guidance and clarity regarding a specific situation. Learning to hear, listen, trust, and heed the gifts of insight may take a little time. Remain open and patient. When you receive guidance, simply act upon it. Don't ponder and analyze it, because your inner critic will pause your progress. Our soul knows and wants what is best for us; you can always trust your soul's guidance.

Healing anchors: Daily life has a way of keeping us busy, delaying, averting, or derailing us from our desired outcomes. When we relapse, we begin to lose faith in our preferred beliefs. Although challenges and setbacks will arise, these challenges strengthen our resolve and guide us in fine-tuning our course of action. Now more than ever, you must exercise unfaltering discipline, believing and trusting in your inner guidance.

Anchors will help you stay strong in your faith and desires. Anchors can be anything, literally. They can be a picture on the wall, a totem, pocket rock, coin, pen, crystal, piece of jewelry, statue, or something you create. An anchor is any item that you assign your promise to, and each time you glance at this anchor you are reminded of your desired outcome, of your greatest trust in yourself, and of your ability to heal your body. It will prompt you to get back on track if you've veered off. It inspires you to keep going, to remain faithful to yourself, and reminds you that you know that healing takes time, that it is okay to feel uncertain at times, but also knowing that you are resolute in your path.

Carefully select something that has meaning to you, and hold it when you're in meditation or prayer, infusing it with your loving energy and highest desired outcome.

Create one anchor for each space you occupy in your home, workspace, and car. Each time your eyes connect with your anchor throughout the day, purposefully take a slow deep breath and connect with the energy of that belief, and smile. Healing anchors are powerful. They inspire us, shift our energy toward hope, and instantaneously connect us to our faith, belief, and trust.

When Pessimism Sneaks In

When you're feeling pessimistic, read through your journal from the beginning, noting how far you've come. Healing takes time; mine took a decade.

Parent your inner child. Write inspirational words, statements, quotes, or declarations on sticky notes, then stick them in places where you will see them frequently—the bathroom mirror, bathroom door, inside the coffee/tea cabinet, the refrigerator, on the ceiling where you first open your eyes each day, etc. Keep them fresh, and change them often. As we upgrade our thoughts and beliefs, so should our reminders and affirmations be upgraded.

Write an "I love" list by jotting down everything you love. Examples: I love me! I love life and all it brings. I love painting. I love reading. I love knitting. I love chocolate. I love cooking. I love walking on the beach. I love gardening. I love spending time in nature. I love my family and friends. I love massage. I love sharing my knowledge. I love spirituality. I love yoga. I love giving. I love reiki. I love meditation. I love experimentation. I love plant medicine. I love swimming. I love snorkeling. I love kayaking. I love people. I love experiencing cultures. I love exploring new foods. I love herbalism. I love breathwork. I love reading the Bible. I love making soap. I love creating jewelry. I love writing. I love easing the suffering of others. I love learning. I love my chickens. I love my cat. I love my parrot. I love all animals. I love creating. I love labyrinths. I love researching. I love traveling. I love fitness. I love feeling great. I love journeying. I love sleeping. I love learning the handpan. I love listening to music. I love philosophy. I love lying in the sun. I love exploring what is beyond. I love walking on the beach. I love feeding the birds. I love sitting still and connecting with all that is. I love I am that I am. I love figuring out how to heal a symptom.

There is so much to feel great about. Illness can sometimes cloud our focus and desires. Let your "I love" list inspire you to refocus your thoughts.

Chapter 4

EXPLORING EMOTIONS

**Your body is an emotional filter and bears the
unmistakable marks of your prevalent emotions.
Emotional disturbances, especially suppressed
emotions, are the causes of all disease.**
—NEVILLE GODDARD

As you explore your emotions, ask for spiritual and emotional help. Calling for help from your understanding of a higher power can be comforting. Consider seeking counseling support from a social worker, therapist, friend, or clergy. I found solitude most beneficial to my progress when working through my feelings. Honoring my emotions was monumental to my healing. What follows is a sample of emotions I experienced and how I navigated them for success.

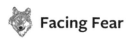 ## Facing Fear

Fear of disease killed more men than disease itself.
—MAHATMA GANDHI

Hearing the words "You have an autoimmune disease," "Your test is positive," or "There's no cure" can create overwhelming fear and paralyzing anxiety. Fear and anxiety are debilitating, preventing us from moving forward toward healing.

Recall that disease is just a *name* given to a set of symptoms; it's *not* a death sentence. Take time to connect with your feelings, beliefs, emotions, and knowledge surrounding this diagnosis. Confronting and clarifying your fear brings awareness and a new, self-reliant, empowering perspective to the situation.

Let the following exercise prompt you to investigate, expand your knowledge, and become your best advocate. Self-inquisition is a potent key to healing. Continually educating yourself about the diagnosis may ease your mind, instill confidence, and empower you to maintain firm boundaries when others challenge your decisions.

 Action: To reduce anxiety, lengthen your exhalations. Try regulating your breath so that your exhale is slower than your inhale. Our heart rate speeds up when we inhale, and upon exhale it slows. Try cyclic breathing, in for a count of four and out for a count of eight or ten, to calm your nervousness.

Journaling: To ease your fears, use the following journaling questions. Answer as many or as few as necessary to create awareness, develop self-reliance, and inspire research. Take your time journaling your responses.

- Hearing the diagnosis, what are you most fearful of? Why are you feeling this way? What knowledge are your fears based on (preliminary research, one doctor's opinion, a relative's experience, etc.)? How can you expand your knowledge (research, speaking to several doctors or others with the disease, etc.)?

- Describe what your fear *feels* like physically and emotionally. Take note of the way hearing that you have this diagnosis is manifesting in your body (tension, insomnia, weakness, etc.), mind (pessimistic thinking, racing or obsessive thoughts, etc.), and emotions (anger, anxiety, depression, etc.). How might these beliefs and feelings contribute to feeling worse or exacerbating the symptoms?

- Is there truly only one outcome for this diagnosis? Have you researched other outcomes aside from what you believe or were told? If not, what are other possible results? (Take time to explore the internet for positive results.)

- Has anyone ever been cured of this disease to date? How did they do it?

- What is your personal belief surrounding this diagnosis? What is the opposite of this belief? What is your desired view?

- How will remaining fearful benefit you?

- How can remaining fearful prevent you from healing? (added stress, insomnia, etc.)

- Are you willing and ready to let go of the fear and adopt an optimistic way of thinking?

- What if you changed this feared outcome? What if you healed yourself?

- What if you took this fear and turned it into positive action steps toward educating yourself and learning how to heal? What would that look like for you? What steps would you take first, second, third, etc.?

Knowledge is the potential power to heal. Expect your doctors to have only some of the answers. They're busy and don't know everything about your illness. The medical community relies upon peer-reviewed research. Consider sharing your research with your medical professionals.

I was obsessed with healing myself. I researched incessantly, documented my findings, and then shared my results with my doctors. I'd print out the studies and bring them to my appointments, asking my physicians if they would support me in trying something I read that had helped someone else. Surprisingly, some of my specialists respected and cautiously supported my decisions. Believe in yourself, assume the best outcome, and be prepared by conducting thorough research and demonstrating where you obtained it. Find a new doctor if your physician disrespects you or disregards your research. You want a team that supports you.

To expand your knowledge, consider some of these research publications and websites:

- National Institutes of Health (NIH)

- Johns Hopkins Hospital

- Mayo Clinic

- The Lancet

- PubMed

- Journal of the American Medical Association (JAMA)
- JAMA Internal Medicine
- The British Medical Journal
- New England Journal of Medicine

Releasing

State aloud and write in your journal: "I release all fear and anything that doesn't support my healing. I create my ideal health now." As stated earlier, use this affirmation or create your own healing affirmations. Then, based on the answers from your journaling exercise, list what you will do to change the feared outcome. As you write, remember that there are no limits; everything is possible. You can heal yourself.

If there are moments of doubt, the moment you catch yourself thinking or speaking negatively, close your eyes and state, "I withdraw that statement," or "cancel that." Reframe the statement into a beneficial one. Then affirm your highest desired belief by repeating the new statement several times.

Example: You think, "Why me? This isn't fair. I don't deserve this." Instead, restate it as, "I am strong, and I am healing my body. I am in control of my health and my future. I am grateful for the gift of healing." Repeat.

 Action: A robust set of affirmations created by Dr. Mikao Usui called the Reiki Principles (*pronounced RAY-kee*) are life-changing and anchored me in my desired beliefs. They comforted me and kept me centered and positive during my healing journey. When I began to feel anxious, fearful, angry, or frustrated, I'd take a moment and do the following:

Get centered in your healing space. Close your eyes, put your hands in prayer, and slowly, deeply inhale through your nose, saying each sentence below silently to yourself, envisioning and sensing the breath and statement filling every cell of your being.

With a slightly open-mouthed exhale, state the same sentence while exhaling the energy of this desired belief into the universe, then repeat each sentence of the Reiki Principles to yourself, and then end the exercise by rereading all of the tenets aloud. Take your time and feel each belief as it becomes yours.

(Abridged)
Just for today, I will not *anger*.
Just for today, I will not *worry*.
Just for today, I will be *grateful for all my blessings*.
Just for today, I will *work with honesty and integrity*.
Just for today, I will be *kind to all living beings*.

**Nothing in life is to be feared;
it is only to be understood.
Now is the time to understand more,
so that we may fear less.
—MARIE CURIE**

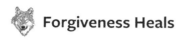

Forgiveness Heals

**Resentment is like drinking poison
and then hoping it will kill your enemies.
—TRADITIONAL SAYING**

Forgiveness is a conscious and intentional decision to release resentment and anger. It does not mean that you forget or excuse an offense. Instead, forgiveness frees *you* from the attachment to the harmful memories.

Anger and resentment are negative emotions that contribute to illness. Forgiveness brings peace of mind and liberates you from the harmful effects of anger and resentment.

I was in my mid-twenties when I was diagnosed with lupus. At that point in my life, I had experienced years of trauma, including leaving home at age 15, homelessness, molestation, anorexia, bulimia, numerous surgeries, the wrong marriage, and a car accident. I had a few people to forgive before I could heal fully. It wasn't an easy process; it took time and was ongoing, yet it was an essential step that paved the way to my healing and freedom.

Journaling: Retreat to your healing space. Before beginning this exercise, light a candle and play your favorite meditative dance music. While standing barefoot, close your eyes and slowly stretch and move your body to the music in a way that makes you feel good. Standing movements help you feel grounded and connected to yourself and get your energy moving. One of my favorite songs to awaken and ground me within before I begin journaling is "Dejemos al Menos Cantos" by Mirabai Ceiba.

Remember to tune into your mind and body during the following exercise. Aside from noting your emotions, take time to feel where these emotions are anchored in your body. For example, you may feel nothing, and that's okay, or you may notice a racing heart, tension in your neck or shoulders, a headache, a pit in your stomach, a compulsion to move your legs, or a sense of needing to escape and run as fast as you can to avoid feeling. Your joints or muscles may begin to ache, or other symptoms may arise. Briefly acknowledge the sensations. Speaking to them, say something loving like, "Ah, that's where you've been hiding. It's safe to come out now. I am here and no longer need protection." Speak to each sensation with love and compassion, just as you would speak to a child. Let them know that it's safe to go now, that you are grateful for their protection but are ready to let go and move on. Remember to breathe slow, chest-expanding breaths as you write, and as you exhale, envision the trapped energy and pain releasing.

 Action: Prepare your sacred space for maximum comfort. Have your journal, a blank notepad, and a pen nearby. Get comfortable in your seat, close your eyes, and place your hands on top of one another at the center of your chest, your heart center. Bring your focus to your breath, slowly inhaling and exhaling, then focus on your hands and feel your heart beating beneath them. Slowly say to yourself, "I love you; I love you so much," several times, and focus on how that makes you feel. Then say, "This forgiveness exercise is for me, because forgiveness is healing." Welcome all of your emotions and feelings.

Now write "Forgiveness is for My Healing" on the top of the notepad sheet. Next, close your eyes and set an intention to write for at least five minutes; continue writing beyond this time if desired. Then, using the following journal prompt, put your pen on the page and write down whatever comes to mind. Do not censor or judge your writing.

Is there anyone that I need to forgive for me to heal my body of _____? (Write the diagnosis or name your pain.)

Repeatedly ask yourself this question until something begins to surface. Sometimes we don't know we need to forgive anyone; instead, we hold onto bad memories and uncomfortable feelings about them, reliving the events in our minds and creating deeper wounds for ourselves. This exercise clarifies if and who we need to forgive for a particular issue. There may be several individuals, just one person, or you may even need to forgive yourself.

Spontaneous writing helps reveal and process painful memories, those stored deep within our body's tissues. Unprocessed emotions, when left to fester, can manifest physically as pain or illness. Automatic writing without forethought unlocks guarded, deep-seated memories.

Forgiveness is for you, not them. You're forgiving their soul of wrongdoing so that you can free yourself of your (conscious or unconscious) pain. Forgiveness doesn't mean you need to see or speak with them; you are doing this for yourself and not them. However, you may decide to let them know that you forgive them whether they've apologized to you or not. Choose to do what feels right for you.

Once you've written everything, read over what you wrote and circle the name(s) of those you will forgive. Select only one name for each session in the next step.

To feel intensely about a wrong without voicing or expressing that feeling is the beginning of disease— dis-ease—in both body and environment.
—NEVILLE GODDARD

Purging

Select one person you circled (alive or transitioned) from the action step above. Close your eyes and envision them, and briefly recall the emotions you felt surrounding them (anger, resentment, fear, etc.). Connect with how that person made you feel, how their actions affected your life and health, and how hurt, angry, sad, ashamed, etc., you were because of their actions.

Then write them a letter expressing everything that needs to be said, such as how they hurt you, what they should have done, how their actions affected your life, etc. Say everything you've always wanted to say but haven't. There are no boundaries; write it all uncensored.

You can also initially use a recording device. Then, while envisioning them, state their name and connect with and express the emotions that bubble up. Shout, use profanity, and describe every feeling, explaining how what they did had long-term effects, what it did to your relationships with others, how what they did affected you long-term, etc.

Your goal is to purge every last emotion regarding this person or event. Say everything as though you are speaking to their soul, and it's hearing you and silently acknowledging the pain inflicted upon you. Then, listen to the recording and type or handwrite a letter from the recording.

Forgiving

When you're ready to forgive their soul, write their name on the top of the paper and explain what you are forgiving them for and why you chose to forgive them.

Example: *I am forgiving you for all of the pain you caused me throughout my life when you _____ . I am forgiving your soul for my healing, to release me of the ties that bind me to you. (Name), I forgive you.*

Then on a separate piece of paper, write a short prayer of forgiveness to them.

Prayer example: *I pray for your peace and forgive your soul for all the pain you have caused me.*

Fire Ceremony

A fire ceremony is a cleansing and transformative ritual that supports the release of emotions from past situations. It can be a roaring fire in a pit, your fireplace, or a small ceramic bowl sitting in your sink where you place the letter after you've lit it.

As the letter burns, intend to let go of the negative attachments and begin a fresh start. You can state, "I am letting all ill will go regarding this person. This fire transforms all negative memories into forgiveness and peace, releasing me of all painful memories, negativity, anger, hatred, and resentment."

Place the letter into the fire, or light it and place it in the bowl. As it burns, state the person's name aloud and your forgiveness prayer. Finish with a silent prayer of gratitude. Then, if you feel called, journal your experience.

Repeat this exercise for each person you are forgiving, or repeat up to this step while collecting your letters and planning a ceremonial forgiveness day where you burn them all one at one time. This is powerful healing work, and I suggest you have a counseling support system available. Consider working with a social worker, spiritual counselor, or psychotherapist.

You can also explore "Ho'oponopono," an ancient Hawaiian forgiveness practice used to release resentment and heal divided families. YouTube has many great Ho'oponopono teachings, or you can research Brandon Bays' deep healing work called *The Journey Method*.

Forgiveness is freeing and supports healing.

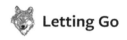 ## Letting Go

**Anything you can't control is for teaching you
how to let go and trust the Universe.**
—Jackson Kiddard

Letting go is empowering; it supports a peaceful state of mind and restores our self-confidence. Letting go is healing.

Healing is a beautiful gift you give yourself; it sets you free. Healing is humbling; it takes strength, decisiveness, commitment, self-love, and revelation. As you free yourself from the confines of an illness, expect that you may need to let go of people and old beliefs. Anticipate feeling melancholic as you heal and release the past. Letting go requires conscious thought followed by action. We heal through our actions, and some efforts require letting go of unhealthy memories and influences.

 Action: In this exercise, you'll practice letting go of memories and people you once cared about who no longer serve your highest good. You may experience a sense of loss of who you were and what was familiar to you. When we lose someone important to us or consciously decide to let someone go, we may need to grieve and mourn our loss. Welcome the range of emotions, and allow yourself time to feel them. Accept that various emotions may come and go in cycles over time. Healing takes courage and time. What awaits you is an expansive lightness in your heart and growing excitement in your spirit—a balance in your emotions and a new and confident perspective of your future.

I created this exercise when I realized that some people close to me didn't support my healing journey, and open and honest communication with them was ineffective. Instead, they were unsupportively stealing my precious time and draining what little energy I had by challenging my decisions. I knew it was vital to change my relationship with them when I realized I was becoming more preoccupied with what they might say or think about my decisions than figuring out how I would heal myself.

To begin, keep a separate "I'm Letting Go" section in your journal. Throughout your healing journey, you should list unsupportive people from whom you want to walk away. Using this list, journal and elaborate on why you chose to let go of these people. Recalling memories and gaining clarity of your *why* helps to ensure this is the right decision for this person. Sometimes a heart-to-heart conversation works best to establish boundaries, and other times it doesn't; journaling will give you the clarity needed to decide your best action.

This list should include people who create negative memories you exhaustingly replay in your mind, creating anxiety, frustration, anger, depression, and hopelessness. Or someone who drains you by doubting or challenging you, because they'll weaken your resolve to heal yourself. Emotions left unchecked manifest as pain and illness and keep us stuck. It's time to gain clarity and let them go.

Letting go of negative people doesn't mean you hate them. It just means that you love yourself.
—TRADITIONAL SAYING

You'll pick one or several people from your list to connect with, feel, and express your emotions surrounding why you are letting them go. You'll let them go with gratitude and a blessing.

Additionally, this exercise can release an old belief; at the end of the activity, you state your up-leveled belief.

This is an imaginary exercise, so make yourself comfortable and have your journal and a pen nearby. Select one event or person from your journal's "I'm Letting Go" section. Close your eyes and recall the hurtful event. Name it—for example, Denying My Ability to Heal, Family Judgment, Jack's Betrayal, etc. State the name aloud. When you're ready to move forward and let go, acknowledge and say aloud that you are letting this person go so you can move forward in your healing. If you're struggling with releasing someone, another way to look at letting go is to approach it as though you're letting them go for a while, not eternally.

Take time to read your journal and recall why you decided to release the bad feelings regarding this person and why you are letting them go. Take a few slow, deep breaths as you connect with the emotions of this decision. Then, tune in to how you feel, taking note of what your body is telling you, of where in your body these emotions reside. For example, is your heart beating faster? Do you feel a lump in your throat or constriction in your chest? Are you nauseous, dizzy, feel weak, exhausted, or are you in pain? *Feel* all of it.

With your eyes still closed, envision blowing the energy of this memory into an imaginary red balloon. As you physically exhale, imagine you are exhaling it into the balloon, expanding it with each exhalation. Each one inflates the balloon a little more, until you decide that it is filled with all the negative emotions surrounding this person. Your goal is to purge every last ounce of unpleasantness you feel about this person or memory. This balloon can be as big or small as you desire.

Next, envision yourself tying off the balloon, and while still holding it, explain aloud why you have chosen to let the person or memory go; explain why it's important to you. For example, you can say something like, "I am letting you go because (you, this memory, etc.) are/is toxic to me. I am letting you go because I realize these feelings keep me stuck and sick. I am letting you go because I no longer wish to feel like I do. I am letting you go because letting go supports my healing. Holding on to this (relationship, belief, etc.) isn't beneficial to my progress." Say all you need to say; speak of the resentment, frustration, anger, unfairness, etc. Then release the balloon.

As you envision the balloon drifting high into the sky, say a prayer or blessing of love, peace, and forgiveness. State aloud that you are doing this to support your healing for your highest and greatest good. Depending on the situation, and only if it applies, thank them for their past involvement in your life, and watch the balloon getting smaller as it slowly drifts higher and higher into the vast universe.

Know that within this balloon are all the emotions, pain, and suffering you experienced, drifting further and further away from you. Watch the balloon ascend until it is no longer visible. Then smile, and through your nose, inhale a slow deep breath, exhale, open your eyes, and journal on this experience and how you feel letting go. Note how your body felt at the beginning of this exercise and again after your release. Spend the rest of the day relaxing and focused on self-care. Repeat this exercise for each memory, person, belief, etc. you decide to let go of.

Sometimes an old memory is awakened, and you'll need to repeat the exercise. You can alter the balloon color, size, and speed as it drifts, or see the balloon pop as it drifts off.

> **Letting go helps us to live in a more peaceful state
> of mind and helps restore our balance.
> It allows others to be responsible for themselves
> and us to take our hands off situations
> that do not belong to us.
> This frees us from unnecessary stress.**
> **—MELODY BEATTIE**

Mastering Emotional Triggers

Unmanaged emotional triggers can begin a chain of undesirable reactions in your mind and body. For example, they can prompt an unhealthy cascade of hormone reactions and lead to anxiety, obsessive thoughts, aggression, depression, inflammation in the body, and dysregulated immune responses.

Mastering emotional triggers supports your healing. When you anticipate the same outcome, you attract the same result. Changing your thoughts hinders the typical response, breaks the chain of events, and changes the outcome. If you can't avoid situations that are known to trigger you, you can control how you react to them.

Knowing what triggers you is the first step to interrupting undesired patterns. Awareness allows you to plan your reaction to future triggers, putting you in control of your emotions. Next, you decide what your desired response is to the stimulus. Finally, conscious awareness of your past reactions enables you to replace them with a response that embodies your preferred character. Stay committed and be patient and nonjudgmental with yourself; change takes practice.

Between an uncontrolled escalation and passivity, there is a demanding road of responsibility that we must follow.
—DOMINIQUE DE VILLEPIN

 Action: Using your journal, begin a section titled "My Desired Reactions to Triggers." First, recall a situation that brought out the worst in you and ask yourself: what is it within me that is being triggered? Where am I feeling this emotion in my body? Why am I *feeling* this way? Why am I *responding* this way? What belief am I holding onto that is no longer serving me and keeps me stuck and reacting this way? What is this situation teaching me about myself? How might my reactions be contributing to my ill health? Finally, what is my highest desired response in this situation in the future?

Next, close your eyes and envision yourself in the triggered situation, see yourself and your undesired reaction, and briefly feel your emotions. Then visualize yourself choosing your desired response to the situation, imagine how you would feel using this response, and immerse yourself in this positive feeling.

Journal about how you felt during the imagined conflict and after you exercised your highest desire. This new response positively shifts your reactive behavior pattern, reinforces boundaries, and empowers you. Instead of flooding your body with long-lasting, damaging stress hormones, you'll nurture yourself with self-control and confidence, freeing yourself from the triggers trap.

Triggers are challenging, especially when we're not feeling well or are tired. If you're triggered and feel challenged to uphold your highest self, excuse yourself from the situation and go to the bathroom to take a moment to compose your thoughts and connect with your most desired reaction. In the future, when you are in the initial stage of a triggered emotion, try closing your eyes while breathing into your heart center and intentionally connect with your highest desired behavior. Stay calm, smile, take a few slow deep breaths and say to yourself, "I am staying calm. I choose my highest desired reaction to this trigger, which is: _____. I remain true to myself and my chosen reaction."

Be patient with yourself; it takes practice to master your emotions! Triggers are an invitation for us to learn and grow. Growth is a process that takes time and commitment, so we can practice our highest desired response. Find what works best for you and do it each time; consistency creates habit.

 ## Fulfilling Unmet Needs

Bitterness never draws us closer to God. Bitterness is a nonproductive, toxic emotion, usually resulting from resentment over unmet needs.
—CRAIG GROESCHEL

Unmet needs are a detriment to our health and well-being, and they fuel illness. Feelings of frustration, agitation, anger, sadness, and despair are distress signals that alert us that something is off-kilter in our life. It is essential to acknowledge and explore these signals when they arise, trace them to their source, and fulfill the need.

When I was initially struggling with lupus, I wanted a loving and supportive community. I wanted help, sympathy, and compassion; after all, I had been diagnosed with a terminal illness, and the doctors had given me five to seven years to live. Instead, I was greeted with judgment and doubt. I was angry, frustrated, and disappointed, and I felt very alone. During this time, I learned that some people couldn't bear to watch my suffering. Instead, they created excuses and distanced themselves or created an unpleasant environment by challenging my decision to find a way to heal, knowing that I wouldn't want them around if they challenged me. They felt most comfortable when they knew the medical community was supporting me because they didn't know how to. Initially, I moaned and groaned to myself and became bitter and judgmental of them. Then I realized that the emotions I felt toward them, or in response to their reactions, weren't going to support my optimistic desired outlook for myself. So, I decided to become my everything; becoming fully self-reliant was my healthiest option.

What are unmet needs, and how do they appear in our lives? When dealing with chronic illness, they can take on such forms as:

- Ineffective healthcare
- Unsupportive living and social environments
- Reduced mobility
- Inability to work/income reduction
- Loneliness

When you connect with your feelings with a loving heart and discover where they arise, you can begin to take steps to fulfill those needs yourself. Self-reliance is empowering and speeds healing.

You can find yourself stuck because of false beliefs and procrastination, and the longer you avoid discovering an unmet need, the longer you will suffer its effects. Exacerbation of an illness can occur from neglecting your needs.

Stop saying you'll do it later, tomorrow, next week. Stop putting others' needs before your own. Don't allow the busyness of perceived obligation to consume you; everything else can wait. You are the most important person in your life. Consciously decide and commit to discovering and fulfilling all of *your* needs.

Discovery is the first step. Often, we don't immediately know *why* we're *feeling* a certain way. We guess and shift blame onto different factors, and then we settle and accept the belief we created as truth. We say, "Maybe it's the food I ate." "I'm irritable because I didn't get enough sleep." "It must be _____ (disease) progressing." "The medication makes me feel _____." During an illness, we become proficient at deflecting and accepting.

 Action: To discover where the symptoms are arising from (the unmet need), you must connect with the symptom or emotion. Sit with it, and have the intention of welcoming it to express and reveal itself to you. Please don't assume you know where the emotion stems from; take time to honor yourself, discover the root cause, and don't brush it off. Your authentic self will always reveal the truth. Let the silence of meditation guide you to peace and clarity.

For example, imagine you're irritable and becoming impatient with someone or something you're doing. To discover where this (feeling/emotion/symptom) arises from, sit comfortably with your hands on your heart center or in prayer. Then close your eyes, take a slow, full breath in, and then slowly exhale; repeat the breath until you feel yourself relaxing and connecting with your higher self (your peaceful, calm self) and ask yourself: "Where is this (feeling/emotion/symptom, describing it with specificity) originating from, and what action steps must I take to satisfy this need for my highest and greatest good?" When you're done posing the question, sit for ten minutes or so, continuing the slow deep breaths, then journal on the experience. The guidance you seek will come either during your meditation, when you journal, when you least expect it, or in your dreams. Sometimes the awareness of the issue is enough to release the undesirable emotion and shift your energy. Other times you will have to create an action plan to initiate the change to fulfill your needs. For more clarity, you can repeat this exercise by asking, "Which step should I take first to facilitate this change?" Give gratitude for the discovery, clarity, and guidance.

Once you've discovered the root cause, act upon fulfilling this unmet need by trusting your higher self. Take time to give love to and nurture yourself. Fulfilling your needs is an act of self-respect and self-love.

 Affirmations: I put my needs before all else. I am the most important person in my life. When my needs are met, I am healthier and happier.

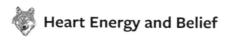

Heart Energy and Belief

Heart-focused, sincere, positive feeling states boost the immune system, while negative emotions can suppress the immune response for up to six hours.

—HEARTMATH INSTITUTE

Envision for a moment the joy of a child frolicking fearlessly in nature; the exuberance, squeals of delight, openness, and trusting heart. That childlike bliss is within you and is another key to healing yourself.

Our hearts become imprisoned by our experiences, emotions, and beliefs. The army of beliefs surrounds the heart in an attempt to protect it from being hurt yet again. In actuality, this army is slowly squeezing us to death. It diminishes our joy and lifeforce energy if we allow it. The peace and freedom we seek are revealed when we let the army retreat.

Aristotle wrote that the soul resides within our hearts. Our soul is the source of our existence, our spark of life. The heart is also where the body's subtle energy system bridges our physical body. We are animated by our life force, aka subtle energy. Chakras are energy centers within our subtle body that act as gatekeepers of our life force energy. As a result, they influence our mental and physical bodies and shape our overall well-being and health. When the body's energy flow is out of balance, this imbalance can contribute to a diseased state of being. Conversely, a healthy energy flow supports balance and harmony in life and health. (This is a brief and simplified explanation of my understanding of our life force energy. I suggest reading Natalie Southgate, Donna Eden, Dr. Bruce Lipton, or Anodea Judith's books about energy and the chakras to learn more.)

Balancing each chakra is equally important. However, a balanced heart chakra supports the immune system, self-love, compassion, shifting beliefs, empathy, and inner peace; it bridges the flow between the physical chakras (root, sacral, solar plexus) and spiritual chakras (throat, third eye, crown), supporting an overall balance of the subtle energy.

I focused on balancing my heart chakra, because the barrage of traumas I experienced in my younger years had caused me to be overprotective in guarding my heart. As a result, I was in apprehensive overdrive, living on high alert at all times, energetically suffocating my life force energy. The energy created by my thoughts, actions, and beliefs negatively influenced the flow of my subtle energy. We are to guard our heart above all else, because everything we do flows from it, but we're not to imprison it. My beliefs were supporting ill health.

Getting the army of unpleasant beliefs surrounding your heart to retreat supports rebalancing. The body positively responds and can heal faster when the heart is in flow with all of life. Let your beliefs heal you.

 Action: You can retreat to your healing space when you begin this practice, but ideally, you'll want to repeat your affirmations throughout each day. As previously mentioned, repeating a statement, mantra, or affirmation supports establishing new beliefs. State the affirmations with conviction. When we proclaim that which we desire for ourselves, we bring it to life. Say them to yourself and state them aloud as often as you wish.

The following affirmations helped me reconnect to a deep sense of love and purpose. Choose affirmations that support what you want to believe and how you want to feel. Consistent repetition facilitates success. Write them on sticky notes and stick them in locations where you'll see them throughout the day. Use a smartphone application with pop-up notifications that allow you to enter your own affirmations. Keep your list at your bedside and recite it each night before you sleep.

We speak what we desire into being. As you state each aloud, focus on and feel the meaning and vibration of each word.

- I welcome new experiences with an open heart.

- I lovingly guard my compassionate heart.

- I am grateful for my loving heart.

- I am grateful for my past experiences.

- Allowing myself to feel love is safe and comforting.

- I am bathed in light and love.

- I inhale and exhale love.

- Each heartbeat circulates love throughout my body.

- I see love all around me.

- I am courageous.

- Love heals me.

- I am filled with gratitude for the love-filled life I'm living.

- I am a beautiful being, and love flows through me.

- I am loved, and I am loveable.

- Healthy boundaries allow me to guard my heart without overprotecting it.

- It is healthy and safe for me to trust myself.

- My heart radiates love and compassion.

- I am always protected.

- I see and focus my thoughts on all of the beauty and goodness in the world.

- I focus my mind on positive thoughts.

- I easily restate unfavorable beliefs into loving, supportive ones.

- I am healed, I am healthy, I am whole.

Chapter 5

HARNESS
HEALING ENERGY

Have you ever felt a surge of positive energy that lifted your spirits or brought a sense of peace? That's the healing energy that surrounds us in countless forms. It's like a hidden treasure waiting to be discovered and harnessed for our well-being. In this chapter, I want to share some exercises that have been instrumental in my healing journey.

Think of these exercises as little adventures into the realm of healing energy. Each one offers a unique opportunity to connect with and tap into the abundant blessings surrounding us. By exploring these practices, you'll find inspiration and discover ways to harness the healing energy that resonates with your soul.

Get ready to feel uplifted, rejuvenated, and truly alive as you embrace the wonders that await you.

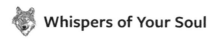 **Whispers of Your Soul**

The Soul always knows what to do to heal itself.
The challenge is to silence the mind.

—CAROLINE MYSS

I call them soul whispers, those blessings of guidance that led me to my victorious healing. How each of us describes or terms this guidance isn't what matters; what does matter is that we listen to the guidance we receive. I'm talking about those wisps of knowingness, where you "just know" or when your "gut" tells you something. Some call it God, or angel whispers; others call it their authentic self, the voice of wisdom, sixth sense, or intuition. What's important is that you take time to honor the gifts of knowledge you are receiving. They may save your life.

Do you listen and trust your soul's guidance? Have you lost connection with your spiritual self, the part of you that is all-knowing and all-loving, guiding your decisions? Do you hear your soul's guidance and doubt the gifts of knowledge you're given? Often, we "hear," doubt, or contemplate them and then disregard them because the message doesn't "fit in" with what we believe to be accurate based on our current beliefs. We may like the message, but it may not fit the societal "norm," so we quickly dismiss it. Your soul's whispers are lovingly nurturing and guiding you toward fulfilling your purpose.

In my experience, its whispers are similar to a domino effect; when I heed a message, another is shared, and so on. On the other hand, if I disregard it, the messages become few and far between, and eventually I stop hearing them. Life became easier when I followed my soul's whispers. Conversely, I struggled when I didn't follow them, and healing was halted. I quickly learned it was in my best interest to trust this guidance.

We all have a lifelong mission to accomplish, and when we're fulfilling it, life is easier; we're happy and healthier. Our soul whispers guide and support us to fulfill our calling.

It takes self-love, conviction, and steadfast courage to heal. Welcome your soul to guide and support you; let it ease your burdens. Take time each day to listen and follow the wisdom of your soul. When you veer off-course, your soul knows how to guide and anchor you back home. Trust your inner knowing, instincts, and intuition; these are your benevolent soul's whispers.

> **Plan time for quiet contemplation or meditation.**
> **Ask your soul to give you information about**
> **your divine greatness. You are your perfect teacher.**
> **—VALERIE HUNT, PH.D.**

Connect. Reflect. Transform. Tap into the energy and wisdom of your soul, and make it a daily practice. Set aside thirty minutes for this exercise by "making an appointment with yourself" and putting it on your calendar. Set the intention to connect with your soul.

Make yourself comfortable in your sacred space and play your favorite meditation music. My favorite music for this exercise is "Healing Presence" by Julie True.

Close your eyes and put your hands on your heart center, the dominant hand on first, as it imparts a sense of calmness, and the palm of your nondominant hand on top.

Take a deep breath in and exhale it slowly, relaxing your shoulders.

Take another deep breath and exhale with a long sigh. *Haaaaaaaa.*

Take another deep breath and exhale it and any tension in your body with a long hum. *Mmmmmmmmm.*

Return to your natural breath. Then, intending to connect with your soul, silently ask the question of your choice from the list below, or one of your own questions. Then repeat, asking it slowly, waiting fifteen seconds or so before you ask again and again, until you hear your soul's guidance. Then, continue questioning to obtain clarity, and give gratitude for the direction.

If you're met with silence after several minutes of patiently waiting for a response, take this time to give gratitude for all the blessings in your life. Attempt to tune in at another time that day. Be gentle, expect nothing, and show appreciation for everything. And know that your guidance may come later in the day when you least expect it. Ask a question of your own or use one of the following:

- Beautiful Soul, what guidance can you share with me today?

- How may I best serve in my life today?

- What is my next best step toward healing, and how best can I fulfill that?

- What can I do for myself today that aligns with my true purpose?

- What is my purpose at this point in my life, and how can I best fulfill this commitment?

After you've given gratitude, sit quietly, bathing in the beauty of your soul's guidance.

Take time to journal about your experience without judging or censoring your writing. Write steps to honor your soul's wisdom, write these plans in your journal, and date the entries.

Simple Joys: Embrace the Little Things

**See the world through the eyes of your inner child.
The eyes that sparkle in awe and amazement
as they see love, magic, and mystery
in the most ordinary things.
—HENNA SOHAIL**

How does joy show up in your life each day? When it does, do you welcome it and take a moment to *feel* how your body reacts to it? Do you show gratitude for it?

Simple pleasures are all around us; they elevate our spirits and feed our souls. Intentionally connect with that which brings you a smile, makes your heart flutter, draws you in, and creates warmth and lightness in your heart every day.

Just as negative thoughts can depress your mood, small joys appreciated each day uplift and strengthen your vitality. For example, simple actions like smiling, laughing, walking in nature, hugging, petting a cat or a dog, or playing with a child release the brain chemicals dopamine and serotonin. These feel-good chemicals are beneficial because they regulate mood and modulate pain, motivating us to repeat the behavior.

Consistent joyful moments sustain and stabilize our mood. When your energy is elevated, you'll likely stay enthused, optimistic, and committed to your healing journey. When you feel crummy, this is a surefire moment to shift your thoughts to something pleasant. I know it's not easy, especially when you are in pain and the medication is depressing your energy and mood, but do it anyway. You'll be happy you did.

> **Self-discipline is the ability to make yourself do
> what you should do, when you should do it,
> whether you feel like it or not.**
>
> **—ELBERT HUBBARD**

Begin the following practice by saying that you won't mention your illness or any of the physical sensations that bother you. I'm not saying to deny how you feel; I'm just suggesting that you redirect your focus. When we redirect our focus toward pleasant things, these small joys crowd out negative sensations such as fatigue and pain. Fill yourself with joy!

Look around you. What do you see in your immediate area that brings you joy? Is it a plant, a pet, a memory from a photograph, a book, wildlife activity outside your window, a song on the radio, a gift, or your vision board? Take time to notice, connect with it, and focus on the feelings this blessing conjures.

- If you're at home, clear clutter; just five minutes of organizing your space can brighten your day.

- Pick some flowers and put a small bouquet in every room.

- Put a pot of water on the stove, add some vanilla or cinnamon, set it on low, and allow the scent to fill the air.

- Play your favorite music and dance around.

- Watch the birds and listen to their sweet songs.

- Read devotions.

- Look in the mirror, give yourself a *big* hug, and tell yourself how proud you are of your steps to heal yourself.

- Plan a dinner for someone special.

- Make a body scrub and give yourself a mini-home spa day.

- Write a poem about joyful moments.
- Call someone and tell them how grateful you are that they are your friend.
- Play an instrument.
- Start a new craft.

If you plan to leave home for the day, consciously seek out simple pleasures and take action without expectation. Actively look for ways to experience and nurture joy, and watch your energy soar!

- Smile, and let your joy shine bright!
- Do a random act of kindness; let someone go before you, hold the door, smile and say something kind.
- Hand out inspirational cards to people you meet in your travels.
- Bring flowers to one of your neighbors.
- Bring the medical staff a special treat on your next visit.
- Share your healing experience with another patient to inspire hope.
- Give someone a genuine compliment. If you notice something, say it.
- Offer to help someone even though you might not feel your best…and watch the pain subside!
- Donate cherished belongings to a charity, knowing they will bring another delight. If you don't use it, share it!

Opportunities for joy are endless; take time to notice, discover, and feel what you enjoy most, and do it often. Often overlooked, simple pleasures cultivate a spirit of joy and gratitude and accelerate your healing.

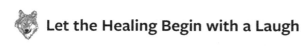

Let the Healing Begin with a Laugh

Your body cannot heal without play.
Your mind cannot heal without laughter.
Your soul cannot heal without joy.
—CATHERINE RIPPERGER FENWICK

It's true! Laughter is one of the best medicines. It energizes and calms us; it releases endorphins, the "feel-good" hormones, and reduces cortisol and epinephrine stress hormones. Norwegian researchers discovered that having a sense of humor is health-protecting. They report that women who scored high on the humor cognitive component scale were less likely to die from a cardiovascular event; both men and women were less likely to die from an infection. Laughing is health-promoting.

So, what did I do to cultivate laughter in my life when I was feeling awful? First, I consciously decided to step away from the stress of daily life; then, I invited laughter to be the impetus that fueled me. Simply put, I engaged in activities that made me laugh. It consisted of watching comedies (25 years ago, I had to rent VHS videos!), engaging with young children, and going to comedy shows. Little by little, my spark of laughter grew into a roaring fire!

You can also welcome more laughter into your life with these ideas as well:

- Purchase a daily joke calendar, and start your day with a funny joke.

- Start your day with a coffee mug that gets you laughing.

- Watch bloopers or funny pet videos.

- Listen to a humorous podcast.

- Write a list of your favorite comedians and comedic actors, search the internet for some of their videos or films, and spend time watching them.

- Call a friend and share the laughter.

- Learn Laughter Yoga, aka Laughter Exercise.

Whatever you choose for your laughter practice, set aside time each day to let go of the seriousness of life and commit to laughing. Invite laughter to become an unconditional sacred practice. Laughter is contagious, so surround yourself with people who love to laugh.

I have been confronted with many difficulties throughout the course of my life, and my country is going through a critical period. But I laugh often, and my laughter is contagious. When people ask me how I find the strength to laugh now, I reply that I am a professional laugher.
—THE DALAI LAMA

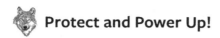

Protect and Power Up!

Energy Medicine puts your health and well-being into your own hands. Your aura learns how to protect you in the increasingly complex situations we encounter today.

—DONNA EDEN

We are energy beings and transmit and receive energy through our body's energy field, aka auric field. This invisible-to-most field of energy surrounds our physical body. It is influenced by our feelings, our thoughts, our health, electromagnetic fields, what we ingest, others around us, and more. Although we may not see the aura surrounding someone, our energy field communicates with it.

Think about someone you know who's warm and welcoming; they're positive, kind, and pleasant to be around, and their upbeat personality positively influences how you feel when you're in their presence. In contrast, someone who's pessimistic and always complaining impacts your energy negatively. After a brief conversation with them, you quickly note a downshift in your energy or an increase in gloomy, negative thoughts. These energetic entanglements play a considerable role in our ability to heal. Living or working with someone negative is a constant drain on our energy and is detrimental to our ability to heal. This passive energy drain is undermining your healing work. You must be mindful of these influences, protect yourself from energy vampires, and recharge your energy.

One day during my lupus healing journey, I felt great. I had energy and wanted to bake some bread, so I went to the supermarket to pick up some yeast. I was excited that I had the desire, time, and energy to bake. I felt fabulous walking into the store, yet only ten minutes later, I walked out feeling fatigued. I felt irritable and perplexed as I sat in my car, wondering what had just happened. How could I feel great one moment and fatigued a few minutes later?

I had been studying Dr. Valerie Hunt's fascinating bioenergy field research at the time, and began to connect the dots. Our physical body has an energy field that picks up and transmits energy. It's an energetic reflection of our thoughts and spiritual, physical, and mental well-being. When we're in close proximity to one another, say standing in checkout lines or sitting in public transportation, our energy fields overlap, and we exchange energies. When we're abundantly energized, healthy, optimistic, well-rested, and know how to recharge ourselves, we can afford to share some of our positive energy with another without it noticeably influencing our own.

The only way I can explain how it drained me so quickly that day is that I was mentally and physically fragile and not abundantly energized or knowledgeable of this phenomenon. To learn more about how your energy field influences your health and healing, you can read the works of Caroline Myss, Donna Eden, or my favorite, Dr. Valerie Hunt.

Using the following techniques, I learned to protect myself and strengthen my field.

Love: The Power Is from Within

The best and most beautiful things in the world cannot be seen or even touched—they must be felt with the heart.
—HELEN KELLER

One of the most profound practices for increasing energy is intentionally radiating unconditional love into the world, intending to ease the suffering of all sentient beings. To engage in this practice, I close my eyes, place my hands on my heart center, and tap into the profound feeling of love within me. With each inhale, I visualize this unconditional loving energy in wave-like pulses, originating from my heart and expanding outward in all directions. And with each exhale, I envision these waves rippling further, embracing the Earth and every living being, enveloping them in love and peace. This practice fills me with energy, peace, patience, and happiness.

Rejuvenate in the Forest

There were months when all I wanted to do was lie in bed. Everything hurt; every joint screamed at me, my head pounded, and my muscles were so stiff that it took every drop of my energy just to get out of bed. All I wanted to do was immerse myself in heat to ease the pain, but I couldn't. I had to get up and go to work. Those were the days I was still living on ibuprofen to ease the pain. The last thing I desired or had energy for was movement; I thought the more I moved, the worse I felt. But what I discovered was that movement is what I needed most! The more I moved, the better I began to feel.

One of my favorite ways to energize is walking in nature. Nature has a way of healing us through its many wonders. Spending time in the forest can reduce stress, improve sleep, and boost our overall well-being. Phytoncides are organic compounds released by trees to defend against insects and fight disease. Research has found that regular inhalation of these compounds can improve the overall functioning of our immune system.

Not in the mood to walk? You can reap the benefits simply by sitting in the forest. I also bring the forest home by snipping some white pine needles and making tea. Pine needle tea has multiple health-promoting properties, and its vitamin C and antioxidant properties are more potent when harvested in the winter.

Not all evergreens are edible—so if you want to incorporate evergreen tea into your diet, make sure you know which needles are edible first. Only consume if you are sure that it is safe.

Water's Gift: Stress Relief and Well-Being Through Negative Ions

This is one time that the word "negative" is welcomed! We all know how vital water is to our survival. But did you know that being in the presence of moving bodies of water, such as cascading waterfalls, a bubbling stream, ocean waves, or even your shower, can make you feel better? Numerous studies have shown the positive effects of exposure to negative ions on stress relief, improved moods, and increased well-being.

Spending time each day to enjoy the sea air helps us relax, restore energy, reduce stress, and improve our overall well-being. Research also demonstrates that these coastal environments increase the production of lymphocytes (white blood cells), which helps protect our bodies from infection and disease. A win-win for autoimmune disease phoenixes!

While I can't say one specific habit healed me, there is no doubt the sea played a major role. When I had lupus, I was drawn to the sea, so much so that I'd plan my days around an ocean visit and winter vacations in the tropics to immerse myself in the sea for hours. I have great respect and honor for the sea. Science tells us that water and minerals cannot pass through our skin membrane, but my body absorbed healing properties from immersing myself in the ocean. I felt more vital and vibrant whenever I came out of the water. The sea undoubtedly contributed to my healing.

Embrace Earth's Healing Energy

Our beautiful planet transmits a healing frequency called the Schumann resonance. It is a natural electromagnetic force that influences our physical and spiritual health. It is a low-frequency signal that increases feelings of well-being. In addition, this frequency links us with the rhythm of nature. According to researchers, it is felt more closely during sunrise and sunset when its intensity increases.

The latest research shows that connecting with Mother Earth, called grounding or earthing, can profoundly impact physical and mental well-being and stabilize our physiology. Earthing or grounding helps restore balance in the body. Earthing techniques include walking barefoot outdoors, swimming in open waters, lying on the ground, and sitting with your back leaning against a tree. With commercial grounding products available for purchase these days, it can be easier to access this connection with the Earth. However, nothing is as powerful as being outside and embracing what Mother Nature offers us.

My favorite way to ground when not swimming is walking barefoot on the beach and then laying on the sand for thirty minutes. When I have more time, I walk to the jetty, lay on the warm rocks, and meditate. It's best in the late afternoon, because the boulders have absorbed the sun's rays all day and are warm and full of healing energy. I'm recharging my human battery with the pulse of the Earth and solar power.

 ## Sunlight and Lupus

I was advised to stay out of the sun when I was diagnosed with lupus, without much explanation other than that the sun could cause symptom flare-ups due to photosensitivity. That advice was highly stressful to me, because I thrive on being out in nature. Initially, I feared the sun as much as the Wicked Witch of the West in the movie *The Wizard of Oz* feared water. I avoided the sun at all costs but became increasingly frustrated with the lack of research supporting this suggestion. At that time, I concluded that this reaction was probably triggered by medications traditionally given to lupus patients, and since I had stopped taking those medications, I decided to venture out.

I've never been a fan of sunblock or store-bought lotions, so I make my own. I had discovered years prior that combining coconut oil and iodine prevented me from getting sunburned, so I mixed up a batch, slathered it on, and took a walk on the beach. I was pleasantly surprised that I didn't get fatigued, as I would most days just walking into a supermarket; in fact, I was energized and exhilarated. I have been enjoying the sunshine for thirty-plus years now without adverse effects.

Note: I was diagnosed with SLE (systemic lupus erythematosus) and discoid lupus after a skin biopsy, but other than an intermittent butterfly rash and hives, I didn't have severe skin reactions. CLE (cutaneous lupus erythematosus) is a form of lupus more associated with severe photosensitive reactions. What is known is that hundreds of drugs are linked to DIL (drug-induced lupus) and that skin rash is one of the most common clinical presentations of DIL. For more, see www.ncbi.nlm.nih.gov/books/NBK441889.

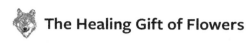

The Healing Gift of Flowers

Healing with the clean, pure, beautiful agents of nature is surely the one method of all which appeals to most of us.
—Dr. Edward Bach

Plants have unique healing frequencies. It's true! The pioneering work of Dr. Edward Bach showed that plants emit vibrational frequencies, which can promote health, well-being, and healing. By understanding the energetic properties of plants, he created a system of natural remedies still used today to treat various ailments. His work is proof that nature has much to offer us when it comes to healing.

The remedies focus on treating a patient's personality, which Bach believed to be the ultimate root cause of disease. Negative thought patterns, feelings, and emotions affect physical and mental health. Each Bach flower remedy is designed to gently correct and balance the vibrations of these negative states so we can live with more ease and vibrant health.

Bach flower remedies are a natural way to address the emotional aspects of illnesses, target the underlying causes, and attempt to correct any psychological blocks that may be causing or aggravating a condition.

In my search for natural remedies, I found great relief from the Bach flower frequency remedies. Mimulus and Sweet Chestnut helped ease the overwhelming, obsessive thoughts and anguish when I first found out I had SLE, and Gentian was a lifesaver for relaxing my mind when I had setbacks and flares. The Rescue Remedy has been a longstanding favorite of mine when I struggle to get a good night's sleep or am anxious about something.

If you are interested in exploring the remedies, I suggest you read one of the many books published by Dr. Bach himself, or visit the Bach Centre website.

 ## Cleansing Your Energy Field

Dry bathing is an energy cleansing practice used by Reiki practitioners and other energy healers. The purpose of dry bathing is to reset and recalibrate your energy field, inviting you to disconnect from people, things, thoughts, emotions, feelings, and situations that cloud your ability to stay balanced.

Incorporating energy bathing into your wellness routine allows you to relax and restore balance and harmony within your body and mind. In addition, this is an excellent practice for shifting from one of your daily tasks to another or when you have experienced an awkward or unsettling interaction or conversation.

Your goal is to work in your energy field approximately three to five inches off your body; some practitioners feel most comfortable touching their body when sweeping, but I prefer clearing my auric field a couple of inches off my body. Do what feels most comfortable for you.

While standing, take a deep breath as you place your right hand up by your left shoulder, approximately three to five inches off your body. As you exhale, sweep downward across your body toward your right hip, then toward the floor in a smooth motion, intending to release the energy toward the ground. You can shake your hand toward the ground like your fingers are wet, and you're shaking water off of them. Again, using your breath, repeat the steps beginning with your left hand on the right shoulder. Then, place your right hand at the left shoulder and sweep down the left arm's energy field, again discharging the swept energy toward the ground, repeating on the right arm.

Awareness is the first step toward protecting your energy. This unseen field has a strong influence on how we feel. How we feel has a powerful impact on health and healing. We tend to blame everything on our fatigue except that which we cannot see. When I struggled with lupus, I'd avoid large stores and crowds because I'd quickly feel exhausted, something I hadn't experienced in the past. I noticed that I felt great after walking outdoors and exhausted while indoors. Initially, I thought it was the lighting or environmental chemicals, including perfumes. I was overly sensitive to everything. Crowds quickly drained me, and nature enlivened me. I was relentless in my quest to determine what I could do to maintain and restore my energy.

 ## Energizing Breath

If you're practicing self-improvement and are minding your thoughts when you notice a shift in your energy or demeanor, take note of those you've just been around, then take steps to restore your energy. In addition to people influencing your energy negatively, note which medications, supplements, and foods negatively affect you, and consider eliminating them. At the beginning of my illness, I took medications to relax my muscles and reduce inflammation and anxiety, which changed my personality and drained my energy. Before I stopped taking them, I found that the following breathwork and visualization recharged me.

You'll be visualizing sunlight streaming in, entering your body and energizing every cell. Take note of how you feel right now, then rate it on a scale of one to five—a five if you're feeling fabulous and a one if you're feeling energy-depleted. When you're done with the breathwork, rate how you feel again. Many times, when we're feeling energy-depleted, it's because we're dehydrated. Have a glass of water next to you to sip when you're finished. Set an intention of feeling energized.

Start by sitting or lying down comfortably and breathing naturally. Close your eyes and imagine the sun high in the sky above you, and then intend it to radiate down into your solar plexus, the space between your belly button and ribcage. With each breath you take, imagine the radiance and warmth of the bright yellow sun combining with your breath and entering and energizing every cell of your body. Feel its heat as it expands throughout your entire body. After you've visually filled yourself with sunshine, thank the sun for this energizing gift.

Next, breathe in through your nose, deepening your inhalation to fill your lungs and expand your chest. When you feel that you can't fill your lungs any further, take one more sip of air and then hold your breath for a count of fifteen seconds. Focus on relaxing your shoulders. Feel the sun's energy infusing every cell of your being, then to a slow count of ten to fifteen, exhale through your mouth, squeezing every last ounce of air out of your lungs. Hold this exhaled breath for another fifteen seconds. Repeat two more times. (Note: You can begin by holding your inhalations and exhalations for five seconds, working your way up to thirty-second cycles over time.)

This breathing routine helps to detoxify, oxygenate, and energize the body. Take note of how you feel on a scale of one to five, compare it to your starting number, and finish drinking the water to hydrate your newly energized cells.

Unlocking Your Body's Healing Potential with Sound

Sound frequency has long been known to have healing properties that can reduce stress, improve sleep, and even help alleviate chronic pain. Sonic alchemy is the use of sound to produce transformative or healing experiences. Using a combination of music, voice, and other sonic elements, sound can change the listener's physical, emotional, and mental states. Sonic alchemy works through resonance—vibratory patterns transferred between the user and their environment.

Sound therapy has been shown to reduce pain and provide spiritual, emotional, and physical healing. For centuries, shamans have used these techniques to connect an individual's inner self or soul with their body and environment. From rhythm-based tribal chants to calming ambient soundscapes, these sonic experiences can take us on a journey deep within our minds so that we can find answers from our innermost being.

I've been fascinated with the healing potential of frequencies since the early 1980s, after reading about Dr. Royal Raymond Rife and Dr. Hulda Clark's research showing that parasites could be destroyed and diseases cured by passing frequencies through the body.

I used the following sound healing techniques during my healing journey. I hope that you enjoy experimenting with them, too.

Solfeggio frequencies

The word "solfeggio" originates from an ancient musical scale practiced by monks in the tenth century, who believed that the vibrational frequencies of each note stimulated specific brainwave states. Among the oldest and most effective forms of sound healing is Gregorian chants—complex choral works that combine the power of music with words to create an atmosphere of peace and relaxation. By combining Gregorian chants and solfeggio frequencies, you can experience deep relaxation and pain reduction. Research has found that these tones can be used to reduce stress levels and even contribute to longer-term health benefits such as increased circulation or improved immune system functioning.

I play solfeggio music in the background during daily activities; it helps create a sense of inner peace and well-being, allowing me to tackle my day with ease, clarity, and focus. You can listen to solfeggio frequencies and Gregorian chants through online music providers such as Pandora, iTunes, Amazon, Spotify, Apple Music, and YouTube.

Harmonizing humming

Vocal toning is a powerful practice that uses the power of one's voice as an alchemical tool for transformation. It assists in healing physical, emotional, mental, and spiritual blocks and brings about lasting change. It helps cultivate awareness within the self. Vocal tools such as humming and chanting lead us on a journey that encourages healing. It allows us to move deep within ourselves to uncover our true essence, beyond the physical body. Voice alchemy enables us to explore our inner voice's potential for healing and transformation.

Humming helps to connect with your body and mind, easing physical, emotional, mental, and spiritual imbalances. From increasing nitric oxide levels to calming negative thoughts, humming has the potential to bring about powerful healing effects.

During my lupus healing journey, there were days I lay in bed, writhing in muscle and joint pain. I lay in bed praying for relief, and one day my prayers were answered. I was guided to hum! I started with a repetitive deep moan-like humming sound and began to feel an easing in the intensity of my pain. I played with the tones, taking deeper breaths and longer hummed exhales, humming at a higher pitch, exhaling the hum as long as my breath would allow. I'd intentionally send the vibrational hum to areas in my body where I had pain; before I knew it, the pain had lessened.

Humming is a powerful tool for healing and relaxation. It has been used for centuries to reduce stress, anxiety, and physical pain. Research suggests that humming can help reduce pain levels in individuals suffering from chronic pain and improve overall mood. This ancient practice is an easy yet effective way to reduce stress, find inner peace, and restore balance within our bodies.

The connection between humming and nitric oxide has been studied extensively in recent years, providing valuable insight into how we can use humming to improve our health. Nitric oxide is an important signaling molecule that helps regulate a range of functions in the body, including immune response, blood flow and clotting, digestion, and communication between cells. Recent studies have shown that humming increases nitric oxide production in the body, leading to improved cardiovascular health, better sleep quality, reduced stress levels, and a more robust immune system.

According to a 2019 study by researchers at the University of Maryland School of Medicine, humming for fifteen to twenty minutes reduces cortisol levels, lowers heart rate and blood pressure, and decreases inflammation. Humming also activates the vagus nerve, which controls heart rate and blood pressure and stimulates the parasympathetic nervous system, helping to induce relaxation, reduce stress, and promote healing.

Give humming a try! The health benefits are limitless. To get started, pick a favorite song and hum along. There's no wrong way to hum. You can hum along with songs you love, make up a tune, hum to match the sound of a piano key, guitar strum, or sound bowl, or hum a sigh of relief. Playing the harmonica is another way to feel the humming vibration throughout your body.

When I had lupus flares, this was my go-to humming practice:

- Begin in a comfortable position and close your eyes. To warm up, slowly inhale a relaxed, full breath in through your nose; then, with lips slightly parted, gently and fully exhale through your mouth with a long *haaaaaaaaa* sound. If you held out a mirror in front of you, you'd see your breath fog it. Repeat this breath three to five times, and remember to exhale each breath fully before you inhale the next.

- Next, you'll say the word "*hum*" in two parts. The first is the *hu*, and the second is a prolonged *mmm* sound as you exhale your breath. Inhale through your nose, and with your lips slightly open, exhale while saying the *hu*, then close your lips and finish exhaling through your nose while saying *mmmmmmmm* for as long as your exhalation allows.

- Repeat this breath for as long as desired, tuning into where you feel the vibrations most in your body. Then return to your natural breath, remain still, and feel how your vibrational energy affects your body.

Keep it simple. This is a relaxed practice; you are not forcefully inhaling or exhaling. As you become comfortable with the humming breath, play around with the tones and vibrations, making them higher or lower pitched or pulsed. Feel them expand throughout your body, and tune in with where you feel the vibration most. Try to direct the hum into areas of pain, and envision and feel the pain dissipating. Your hum creates a healing vibration unlike any other.

Singing bowls and frame drums

At the height of my lupus journey, there were many days when the pain was deep within my body, and neither heat nor massage would alleviate it. I was determined to find a way to relieve the pain without taking medication, and I began experimenting with handheld drums and singing bowls.

Singing bowls have been used for centuries to promote healing, relaxation, and energy balance in the body. These bowls can take you away from the everyday hustle and bustle of life and usher you into deep relaxation. When held near the body and struck with a mallet, the sound waves generated by striking them penetrate deeply into our cells, improving circulation, reducing stress, and helping to relieve pain. In addition, their harmonious sounds open up our intuition and spiritually awaken us on an energetic level, making it easier for us to focus on healing ourselves.

Buddhist and other Eastern healers have used Tibetan massage bowls for centuries to help people heal. The process is based on the powerful healing properties of sound therapy, derived from ancient principles. The use of these unique massage bowls to facilitate healing involves placing them on various acupressure points on the body.

I had a couple of small bowls I could play while holding them in my hand. Listening, I was immediately transported to a place of peace and tranquility. Later I purchased heavier bowls designed to be played on or next to my body. When I struck these bowls with a soft mallet, I felt their powerful vibration permeate deep within my body. Each time the mallet tapped the bowl, I'd feel another layer of tension dissipate until the pain was no longer there. These bowls were a lifesaver. I'd keep a couple at my bedside for ease of use and grab them instead of ibuprofen. Not only did they relieve my pain, but they also brought me peace and helped me fall asleep easily.

In my quest to heal, I also attended drumming circles and discovered the healing power of the frame drum. Handheld drums can be used for healing by using the drum's rhythmic vibrations to induce relaxation. The rhythmic pulsing of a frame drum helps calm the mind, induces relaxation, and reduces stress levels creating inner balance and harmony.

First, I play the drum around me to clear and enliven the energy in the field around me. While standing, I take a few slow deep breaths and set an intention to cleanse my energy field. Then, using my frame drum and a felted beater stick, I hold the handle on the back of the drum with my nondominant hand and gently tap the drum a couple of times eight to ten inches above the crown of my head and slowly move downward while tapping in a straight line in the front of my body, using the line of the chakras (third eye, throat, heart center, solar plexus, sacral, and root) as my guide. Then I play the drum toward my feet; then working in reverse order, I return to my crown and repeat playing the drum downward on both sides of my body in the same manner. If I have a buddy, I ask them to drum down the back side, then proceed with the following. (Use the following steps as a general guideline; as you drum, allow your inner guide to lead you.)

- Using your sacred space, sit or stand comfortably and set an intention to heal, release tension, reduce pain, or relax. Breathe naturally.

- Close your eyes and hold the handle of the frame drum comfortably in front of you with your nondominant hand.

- Gently tap the drum using a felted beater stick with your other hand.

- Feel the drum's vibration as it permeates your body. Experiment with the drum's vibrations, playing it sideways or focusing the bottom of the drum toward your body.

- Then move the drum so that it's eight to ten inches above areas of pain or tightness, and play it as you are called to; you can tap it slowly, softly, loudly, or create a rhythmic beat. Feel what your body is asking for and enjoy the communication and sensations. Have fun with it. If you feel like dancing to the rhythm, do it!

Another option is to have someone play the drum for you. As you lay on your back, ask them to play the drum beginning at the bottoms of your feet and then slowly over your legs, hips, belly, chest, neck, and crown, then reverse, ending at your feet again. Ask them to focus on areas of pain or tightness, to play slower, faster, etc. When they're done drumming on the front side of your body, turn over and ask them to repeat on your backside.

Remo makes an excellent and inexpensive frame drum. If you're like me and want to learn more, YouTube has several instructional videos under frame or Reiki drumming.

Chapter *6*

HEALING WITH MOVEMENT & MODALITIES

Gentle reminder: Please get your doctor's approval before implementing my suggestions. What helped me might cause a flare for you.

My physical protocol took me years of trial and error. Finally, in desperation to survive, I researched and explored hundreds of topics, implemented various diets, and spent exorbitantly on supplements, hoping for a miracle cure.

I touched on the importance of movement in Chapter 5. In this chapter, I share more of my story and suggestions that contributed to the incremental and compounded healing that took place in my body.

If you try any suggestions, please listen to your body and honor its feedback. If something doesn't feel in alignment with your healing, don't do it. Self-love is tuning into how your body feels and glorifying it; lovingly honoring it sends a powerful message of love and respect.

Find Your Morning Flow

Starting each day with a mindful and gentle approach to movement can significantly impact the rest of your day. Allowing yourself enough time in the morning to ease into the day also sets you up for better mental and emotional resilience.

Daily stretching helps you become more aware of your body and its limitations and creates a space to practice mindfulness and gratitude. Adding positivity to your daily stretches can make a world of difference to your mental and physical state. Giving thanks each day while being intentional with every stretch can cultivate a deeper sense of positivity within yourself. Even something as simple as focusing on one positive quality while stretching can be a source of motivation and joy. Doing so can bring an extra layer of positivity to the activity, creating an opportunity for further connection between body and soul.

As you stretch, take a moment to appreciate the small things in life while considering what specific area of life you are incredibly grateful for and why. Tackling an autoimmune condition can be daunting, but focusing on the good in life—no matter how small— profoundly impacts our outlook for the rest of the day.

Before retiring in the evening, place a large glass of water, a pen, and a journal at your bedside. When you wake in the morning, begin your day by sipping the water while you recall three things you are grateful for. Then, in your journal, list them and elaborate on why you are thankful for them. This connects you with your gratitude on a deeper level. Sit on the side of the bed, take a couple of slow, deep, belly- and chest-expanding breaths, and slowly exhale them. The rest of your movements should be accompanied by conscious breathing and remembering to connect with your feelings of gratitude. This practice hydrates our body, reminds us of how fortunate we are, tunes us into feeling, and balances our thoughts by focusing on what brings joy and satisfaction. These powerful moments help us feel rejuvenated as we start each new day!

Next, awaken your spine by putting your feet firmly on the floor, with the back of your knees touching the edge of the bed, supporting you so you don't fall forward. Then fold your torso over your knees, dangling your arms at your side. Lean forward as far as is comfortable, but know that it may initially feel very tight. Mindfully connect with and feel the stretching of your spine, then slowly sit upright and softly hold the right side of your head with the left hand just above your right ear. Slowly and gently tilt toward the opposite shoulder (don't force it), gently stretching your neck muscles, drop your shoulders if they should come upward, then repeat the stretch on the other side.

Sit straight with your head centered and face forward. Move your chin toward your neck, and hold it for a count of ten. You should feel a gentle stretch to the back of your neck. To envision what I'm referring to, think of jutting your chin and neck forward like a turtle does when it comes out of its shell, then retracting inward until you can't retract further and holding it there as you count to ten. Next, return your head and neck to your neutral center, bring your shoulders up toward your ears, and hold for a count of ten; then slowly rotate them in a circle, forward, downward, and backward a couple of times; then rotate in the opposite direction.

Next, clasp your hands behind your lower back, resting your hands on the bed by your buttocks; this stretches your shoulders backward and opens your chest. Hold this position for a count of ten, then release your clasp, bring your hands in front of you, and then stretch your arms up over your head for a wrist stretch, rotating between facing your palms and the back of the hand toward the ceiling for a count of ten.

Note: **You should skip the following step if you feel lightheaded, have hypertension, or your doctor has advised you against inverting.** Lastly, stand with your legs shoulder width apart, gently fold your body forward, and hang with your fingertips toward the floor, feeling a gentle stretch for as long as you feel comfortable. Then slowly stand upright, smile, drink the rest of your water, make your bed, and begin your day.

Even when facing the challenges of an autoimmune disease, beginning each day with a task accomplished can do wonders for physical, mental, and emotional well-being. It will give you a sense of accomplishment and satisfaction and set the tone for the rest of your day.

> **If you make your bed every morning,**
> **you will have accomplished the first task of the day.**
> **It will give you a small sense of pride, and it will encourage**
> **you to do another task and another and another.**
> **—NAVAL ADMIRAL WILLIAM H. MCRAVEN**

Engaging in prolonged bed rest or extended periods of sitting, which compresses our blood vessels, can result in reduced blood circulation and hinder the proper functioning of our lymphatic system. This may lead to numbness, tingling, and an elevated risk of blood clots while also affecting lymph flow, weakening the immune response, and possibly causing fluid retention and swelling in the affected areas.

Both lupus and the traditional medications prescribed to ease the symptoms have a way of dispiriting and demotivating us. Where we once worked out in the gym for an hour, we can barely muster up the desire or energy to walk to the mailbox—so I created a habit of moving and doing breathwork every waking hour. I set a timer and committed to getting up and moving in some form. These movements eased my pain, uplifted my mood, and inspired me to stay on the healing path.

A few minutes each hour adds up to thirty minutes of movement daily. An inactive body becomes stiff and painful and exacerbates lupus symptoms. Exercise can reduce symptoms by reducing stiffness, improving joint mobility, and increasing energy. Setting an hourly timer on your watch or phone reminds you to get up and move. It only takes a few minutes to invigorate your body.

Lupus-friendly Movement Tips

When I had lupus, I had days where I felt like every muscle was contracted, causing inflammation to every organ in my body. I was stiff and always felt pain somewhere in my body. My pain loved to rotate and refer pain elsewhere. My morning stretching routine kickstarted my day, but I wanted medication-free long-term relief. Restorative and yin styles of yoga were the most beneficial exercises that gave me long-term relief and increased my flexibility without experiencing the rebound pain I'd feel for days following minor activity. These gentle yoga movements were a blessing.

The key to movement lies in being gentle, listening to your body, staying hydrated, and embracing the understanding that regular exercise brings incredible benefits to the psyche, including stress reduction, improved mood, enhanced mental clarity, anxiety relief, boosted self-esteem, better sleep, and increased resilience. While shifting focus from past painful experiences (the rebound pain and fatigue we experienced with lupus following exercise in the past) may be challenging, directing our thoughts toward what we do want instead of what we don't can somehow alter the outcome. Healing is often difficult to articulate, but consistently focusing on the positive benefits is what truly nurtures our well-being day by day.

Yoga

Hire a yoga teacher to teach you floor or chair poses, or view poses specific to your ailment on YouTube. Be sure to find a certified yoga instructor or licensed physical therapist to avoid harming yourself. As mentioned above, yin and restorative yoga are most beneficial for relieving pain and distress.

- *Yin yoga* is a type of yoga that focuses on targeting the connective tissue, or fascia and ligaments—those inner parts of us that lupus so lovingly introduced us to and makes us aware of each day. Unlike more active styles of yoga, such as vinyasa or ashtanga, yin yoga focuses on slower and longer-held poses. These poses allow us to access the deep layers of tissue that aren't accessible during fast-paced poses. By allowing us to stretch these layers of tissue, we can gain greater flexibility and ease the pain. As well as being low impact, the poses bring balance and harmony to the body's energy system, inducing a calming effect on the mind and body that can help combat fatigue.

- *Restorative yoga* helps to relieve stress-related ailments such as pain, soreness, and inflammation by bringing awareness to the breath, stilling the mind, and intentionally surrendering into deep relaxation. During each pose, we can practice finding peace within to release physical or emotional tension. Through this deep mind-body release, we can unlock inner peace by fostering rejuvenation on all levels.

- *Yoga nidra* isn't a movement practice, but it still belongs here with its sister forms of yoga. It's a powerful and ancient yogic technique that can recharge the body during the day and unwind the body at night. It's a relaxation practice that calms the mind and body, creating deep peace and stillness. I struggled to get a good night's sleep many nights, only to find that insomnia exacerbated my pain and agitation the following day and made work almost impossible. Yoga nidra to the rescue! I loved this practice for going off to sleep at night and during the day to recharge me when I was exhausted. Yoga nidra is a great way to melt away stress and rejuvenate daily! Yoga nidra and meditation with some aromatherapy were part of my nightly routine, helping me relax and unwind my mind and body.

Foam roller

My neck, chest, back, and shoulders were always tight when I had SLE. I discovered lying on a four-foot-long foam roller a lifesaving pain reliever, and I still use it today after a long day at my desk to improve my posture through targeted stretching of tight chest muscles.

It alleviates pain and supports you while you're holding yin yoga floor poses. The rollers are inexpensive; search online for a foam or physio roller. Also, check YouTube for foam rolling or foam roller lymphatic massage routines created by trained professionals.

Swimming

I love being near water and find swimming in the sea physically and emotionally healing. Swimming helped me improve my physical strength, reduced inflammation and pain, and was easy on my joints. I always felt uplifted and energized after I spent time in the ocean. Aside from the negative ions and Earth's gift of the Schumann resonances, I knew there was a significant connection between my feeling fabulous and swimming. I believe my body naturally absorbed the nutrients needed to heal from the ocean. No matter how many vitamins and minerals I ingested, I never felt as rejuvenated as I did after swimming in the sea. Like how skin patches administer medication, my body drank what it needed from the ocean. Nature is healing; knowing and listening to your body's subtle messages is vital. My body craved the sea like some of us crave sugar. I've mentioned this before, but it's important to note again that no single thing healed my body by itself. My body knew what it needed to heal and gave me cues. I tuned in, listened, and had faith, and it slowly healed.

Lupus can deteriorate our body if we allow it to. It's a cyclical trickster. One day you're feeling fabulous and want to do everything; the next five days, you're hugging your pillow because you enjoyed an afternoon walk. There were weeks I lay miserably in bed, too fatigued and riddled with pain to want to do anything. The longer I was immobile, the greater my fatigue and discomfort. You might think resting alleviates the pain and inflammation, but you quickly discover that lying around creates new aches and pains, a toxic body, and a depressed mood. It was a complex cycle to break. I was desperate and would try anything to get some relief, but I refused to poison myself with medications. I never gave up hope. Each time I tried something new, I'd speak to it with hope and positivity, and I'd hold this belief and vision even when I had rebound pain. For example, I'd say, "You're going to help me heal my body. I trust that over time you're going to help me feel better and better each day. Thank you for contributing to my healing. I am so grateful I discovered you." I knew immobility was worse for me than gentle movement, so I kept trying new things and rotating them throughout the week.

I discovered several pieces of equipment that supported me throughout my healing journey. They were especially beneficial when I had flares. After I'd finished any of the following, I'd drink a 16- to 20-ounce glass of water to hydrate my body.

Stretch ropes or straps

These bands are compact and practical for stretching and strength training and come with either a booklet or poster of exercise suggestions. You can Google either stretch rope or stretch strap. Most of my fire spots of pain were in my shoulders and neck, and these straps helped to relieve the tension.

Tennis balls

I've used tennis balls to ease pain in my back, especially for spots I couldn't reach. I place the ball on a wall and then gently lean the ball on the pain point while squatting to relieve the blocked energy in the back muscle and strengthen my legs. You can place the ball on a wall or the floor, lean on it, then gently move it from side to side or in a circular motion, being careful to avoid putting any pressure on your spine. If the pressure is too much, you can try the exercise lying on your bed or using a softer ball. Remember to use slow deep breaths when releasing tension.

Isometric exercises

Simple exercises for just a few minutes daily can relieve pain and strengthen muscles. The activities involve static contraction of a muscle without movement of a joint. Your physical therapist can develop a program specific to your needs, or you can search on You-Tube for isometric exercises taught by a physical therapist.

Conscious breathwork

Taking a minute or longer to focus on breathing shifts your energy and mood and oxygenates your blood. Most of us take very shallow breaths all day long. The deeper the inhalation, the better. Inhale a deep breath and hold it for eight to ten seconds, then slowly release it for the exact count, increasing the count with each consecutive breath. Be conscious of areas where you might be holding muscle tension as you do the breathwork and focus on sending the breath there, releasing tension and relaxing the muscle.

Inversion table

Each time I lay on the inversion table, I felt expansiveness and relief from the restrictive tightness throughout my legs, hips, back, neck, and abdomen. Such a table has varying degrees of inversion, and I'd start on the lowest grade and gradually invert to sixty degrees. I'd hold the sixty-degree inversion for three to five minutes with my eyes closed while taking slow deep breaths and envisioning the elongation of my body's tight fibers. The tightness unraveled, and the muscles relaxed.

Alongside my battle with lupus, I also endured the challenges of endometriosis, polycystic ovary disease, and extensive abdominal adhesions, leading to multiple surgeries over several years. Determined to break this cycle, I found a lifeline in inversion therapy, which was a game-changer for both my lupus-related muscle pain and my abdominal adhesions. Each abdominal surgery aimed to address one issue but resulted in post-surgical scarring and adhesions, causing my organs to bind together, leading to digestive problems and excruciating pain. However, as I embraced inversion, the weight of my body gently eased the constriction of these adhesions, allowing them to stretch and unravel, providing much-needed relief.

Feet on the wall

In my search for relief from leg swelling, I discovered and fell in love with putting my legs up on the wall. First, I'd shower, then apply some coconut oil on my feet and legs, gently massaging to help get the fluid moving; then I'd lay on the floor and put my legs up on the wall while I listened to relaxing music and meditated.

Vibration plate

Every morning, I dedicate ten minutes to using a vibration plate, and incorporate it into my daily routine at various times throughout the day. A vibration plate is a fitness device with a vibrating platform. When a person stands, sits, or exercises on the platform, it transmits vibrations throughout the body. These vibrations cause muscles to contract, simulating the effects of exercise and providing various potential health and fitness benefits.

The rapid vibrations from the platform cause muscle contractions, which can assist in pumping lymph fluid through the lymphatic vessels, promoting better circulation and removing waste products and toxins from the body. This can contribute to a healthier lymphatic system and enhance the body's immune response.

I prefer standing on it, but one can benefit from sitting on the plate or sitting in a chair and placing their feet on it. It revitalizes the body, alleviates aches and tension, and reduces swelling. In addition to helping move lymphatic fluid, it prevents poor circulation from sitting for long hours.

Chi machine

Akin to a vibration plate, a chi machine stimulates the lymphatic system. A chi machine is a passive exercise device that promotes relaxation, improves circulation, and boosts the flow of "chi" or energy in the body. It is also known as a "swing machine" or "passive aerobic exerciser." The chi machine typically consists of a padded platform where you lie down with your ankles resting on a footrest.

Once you switch on the machine, it moves your feet from side to side in a gentle swaying motion. This movement is designed to mimic the motion of a fish swimming, and it is believed to stimulate the body's natural energy flow. The elevation of the legs and side-to-side movement of the foot cradle gently shakes the body, while vibrating and emitting infrared heat is profoundly relaxing. Both the vibration plate and the chi machine become your allies on days when you might not feel like moving, providing a gentle and enjoyable way to invigorate your body.

Mini-trampoline/rebounder

Using mini-trampolines can stimulate the lymphatic system, activate muscles, improve circulation and oxygenation, enhance balance, and heat the body. Initially, this was challenging because it felt jarring on my joints; so I'd stand on it and gently bounce for five or ten minutes, and then slowly worked up to jumping. As I began to feel stronger, I'd put on some music and gently jump for a couple of songs to work up a sweat, increasing circulation and lymph movement in my body.

Sauna

Before being diagnosed with lupus, I was an avid cycler and aerobics lover, spending most of my free time at the gym. Some said that I was addicted to exercise. I think I was addicted to endorphins and sweating! When I had lupus, I missed the gym and knew my body wanted to sweat. So, I purchased a plastic sweat suit and wrapped myself in a heating blanket. It wasn't the same as working out, but it did help me perspire. Later, I purchased an at-home portable sauna to sit in while a small pot of distilled water released steam. It was delightful for relieving stiffness and muscle pain, and I'd sleep like a baby.

An interesting sidenote: because I often experienced considerable fatigue after my morning shower, I decided to use the sauna just before going to bed to promote a better night's sleep. My body detective brain figured out that my morning shower fatigue could have been caused by low blood pressure, dehydration, or off-gassing of chlorine. Interestingly, I didn't feel the same overwhelming fatigue following the sauna!

I always have a tall glass of water before and after my saunas to support detoxification and hydration. The first glass has a small pinch of sea salt. Adding a pinch of sea salt to the water before a sauna session offers benefits such as improved hydration, enhanced perspiration, and reduced fatigue associated with low blood pressure. It also provides electrolytes, essential minerals such as sodium, potassium, magnesium, and calcium, which are naturally found in seawater. When sea salt dissolves in water, it releases these electrolytes, providing vital support for fluid balance, nerve function, muscle contractions, and overall cellular activity in the body.

Please remember the importance of knowing your body and seeking guidance from a healthcare professional before incorporating sea salt into your diet, especially if you have medical conditions like lupus nephritis or hypertension. Your health needs are unique, and consulting with an expert will help you make informed decisions for your overall well-being.

Pulsed electromagnetic field (PEMF) mat

During my relentless research to heal myself, I discovered PEMF. When I learned that pulsed electromagnetic field therapy accelerated healing by using magnetic energy to reduce inflammation, increase circulation, improve range of motion and flexibility, and flush toxins, I had to buy one.

PEMF mats are non-invasive devices that transmit low-frequency, low-intensity electromagnetic pulses into the body. These pulses create a natural magnetic field that helps repair damaged tissues and organs due to inflammation, trauma, or other physical issues. PEMF therapy is utilized globally in various settings, including medical facilities, sports medicine, physical therapy clinics, veterinary medicine, and wellness centers. Its benefits include pain management, wound healing, post-surgery recovery, rehabilitation, and overall well-being. Although scientific research is ongoing, PEMF therapy has gained recognition for its non-invasive nature and potential health benefits.

The PEMF mats didn't come cheap, but I was determined to heal myself. When the docs gave me a life expectancy of five to seven years max, I knew healing was my only option, and I committed myself to pave the way at any cost. I devoted an entire decade to conquering this illness, allowing me to spread my expenses over time. I realize not everyone reading this can rush out and buy all the items mentioned in my book—it wasn't feasible for me, either. My focus was twofold: first, to keep living, and then to truly flourish. So, if you're reading this and contemplating trying something that seems too ambitious, don't let financial concerns hold you back; find a way to make it a reality.

For instance, if you're considering trying a PEMF mat, consider experiencing a session at a health and wellness center, physical therapy clinic or spa, or rent a unit. My favorite unit is the QRS. You can learn more about their system, research and benefits at https://www.qrs.com/.

Quantum biofeedback system

Our bodies are intricate networks of energy, with vital currents flowing through every cell and organ, intimately linked to our emotions and thoughts. The quality of this flow, whether unimpeded or restricted, reflects the complex dance of our body-mind intelligence. Quantum biofeedback sheds light on this dynamic by assessing subtle energetic imbalances, revealing hidden stressors, inner conflicts, and blockages. Prolonged stress disrupts this delicate energy flow, creating imbalances that can pave the way for illness. Everything vibrates—our thoughts, emotions, even our organs and cells. This energy extends beyond the physical, forming an auric field that surrounds our bodies. The biofeedback program delves into this energetic realm, recognizing and cataloging unique energy signatures. Through galvanic skin pads, the system communicates with our energy field, generating a detailed report of energetic stressors impacting us. This information allows for the precise delivery of harmonizing frequencies, gently restoring balance and promoting a sense of calm. Initially, I approached quantum biofeedback with cautious optimism. But after each session, I felt a tangible shift, a lightness that gradually peeled away the layers of stress, revealing the "old me" beneath. Months of research—sifting through scholarly articles, reviewing testimonials, and even exploring skeptic perspectives—preceded my decision to invest in this technology. Looking back, it was one of the most transformative health decisions I've made. While there may be aspects of healing that science cannot yet fully explain, I'm content to embrace the profound positive impact it has had on my life.

Chapter 7

BREAKING
THE CYCLE

In addition to having lupus, I had relentless pain from abdominal adhesions resulting from endometriosis, surgeries for polycystic ovary disease, incisional hernia repairs, laparotomies, ectopic pregnancies, fallopian tube reconstruction, and multiple adhesion removal procedures. I fell into a cycle I was desperate to break: the surgeries created an overgrowth of candida, more adhesions, and pain; the adhesions caused constipation, more toxicity and pain; the debilitating pain contributed to a lack of exercise; fatigue and exhaustion contributed to poor dietary habits, which resulted in vitamin and mineral deficiencies.

I concluded that I had to avoid surgery to heal fully, which meant I had to figure out how to break the cycle.

Systemic Enzymes for Eliminating Adhesions

While healing from lupus, I was simultaneously researching to find a cure for eliminating abdominal adhesions, as I had had more surgeries than I care to recount to remove adhesions from my bowel, uterus, and bladder. My first operation was at age 15 for an ovarian cyst; my last was in my early forties for an incisional hernia. I lost count, but it was close to 30 operations in 25 years. Each surgery for adhesion removal gave me approximately six to nine months of reduced pain. Although I had temporary relief, each surgery created more adhesions, gut dysbiosis, pain, and a weakened immune system. I wanted permanent healing.

I researched and discovered a systemic enzyme, a medication used in Europe and Japan for dissolving arterial plaque and reducing inflammation. I wondered why there wasn't any published research on dissolving adhesions, and I decided I wanted to try it to see if it would lessen my pain. By this time, I had suffered crippling abdominal pain for over ten years. I was desperate for a solution to live pain-free and keep me out of the hospital. Intuitively, I knew that there was an association between lupus flares and surgeries. I thought if I could eliminate the problem that kept me returning to the hospital, perhaps I could heal lupus too. I focused on adhesions and discovered that endometriosis was their primary cause. I'd already had several surgeries to snip apart the adhesions that glued some of my organs to one another, but the pain and adhesions always returned.

I found the top adhesion removal specialist in Pennsylvania, Dr. Harry Reich. He had been having great success removing adhesions and endometrial tissue while reducing post-surgical adhesion formation. I was hopeful. I read every article and post in his discussion group and scheduled my surgery.

Before proceeding with this surgery, I first wanted to try the enzyme to see if it would reduce my pain and adhesions. If this enzyme could dissolve arterial plaque, might it dissolve adhesions too? I had high hopes that my theory would prove true. I believed it was the solution to end my suffering. Fortunately, in the United States, it's an over-the-counter supplement.

I printed the research and brought it to my cardiologist. I wanted his opinion as it was a medication used in Germany and Japan for cardiac patients, and I didn't want to cause harm to my body. I wanted to know if he felt it was safe for me to take it to break down adhesions. My cardiologist gave me the go-ahead as long as I promised to stop taking it at least one month before surgery, because he was concerned it might affect blood clotting. I was ecstatic!

I diligently took it and began to feel a lot better. Aside from having less pain, I had more energy and felt like my old self was returning. However, I had the procedure in the fall because I still had some pain.

In preparation for the surgery, I had to provide my past operative records to the surgeon. My prior surgeries took several hours for doctors to cut through layers of adhesions before being able to access my organs. Based on my prior operative reports, he booked the operating room for six hours. Surprisingly, he completed my procedure in one hour and fifteen minutes. I had very few adhesions and several endometrial implants. Having little scar tissue to remove was a huge win; the enzyme had worked! I knew I was onto something.

Now that I had this surgery behind me, I focused on colon health. I prophylactically restarted the enzyme. My goal was to prevent postoperative adhesion formation; in the past, I postoperatively formed adhesions that loved to connect my organs together. I decided to deviate from how I had recovered in the past to see if it made a difference in healing. So, instead of taking the pain medicine codeine, I only took the enzyme, which is a potent anti-inflammatory.

During my recovery time, I studied research on the role that diet plays in endometriosis, PCOD, and candida, and how water fasting (drinking only water) and intermittent fasting (eating only during certain hours of the day) support healing. I began water fasting every Monday for twenty-four hours, sometimes longer. Then, I slowly transitioned to a whole-food, mostly plant-based diet with added chicken or fish a couple of times a week. Many anti-candida diets are intensely restrictive, eliminating grains, legumes, fruit sugars, etc. I tried to follow them at first, but eventually listened to my body for direction instead. It was more important to me to listen and nurture my body with whole foods, including fruits and grains, than to follow a strict restrictive diet.

I introduced green smoothies of kale or spinach, with half of a banana, berries, avocado, hemp, pumpkin, or chia seeds, into my daily meal plan and would drink them twice daily. It was a slow shift to the freshest organic produce I could source. Twice a week, I'd bottle up various juices, including some of the pulp, using kale, spinach, celery, cucumber, beet, parsley, cilantro, lemon, green apple, pineapple, carrots, pears, etc., making it easy to grab on the go. The leftover skins of pineapple and juicer pulp were used to create an electrolyte drink I'd take on my walks.

I grew some of my food and joined a local organic farm co-op. In the wintertime, I ran an organic food co-op out of my garage. Eventually, I raised layer hens for eggs and became a beekeeper. The more I could control what I put into my body, the better.

Instead of adhering to yet another trendy diet that promised miraculous healing, my journey to recovery was a profound shift towards mindful living and a deep connection with the food I consumed. Through intermittent water fasting, transitioning to a balanced, whole-food diet, and embracing the nourishment of green smoothies and homemade juices, I found a path to wellness that allowed me to listen to my body's needs and nurture it with love and care.

 ## Balancing Hormones and Restoring Gut Health

For years, the adhesions and candida contributed to my colon not functioning efficiently. As a result, I had chronic constipation, fatigue, brain fog, irritability, and abdominal pain. In addition, constipation prevents the elimination of waste, including estrogen, which can be reabsorbed by the body and contribute to hormonal imbalances, contributing to endometriosis and PCOD. I thought if I could stop this cycle, I'd be on my path to recovery.

I increased my water intake, exercised most days (I share specific movements I did in Chapter 6), supported lymphatic drainage, and added fiber to my diet. Fiber helps eliminate excess estrogen from the body by binding to it in the digestive tract, carrying the excess out of the body through bowel movements. Additionally, fiber helps maintain healthy gut bacteria. A healthy gut microbiome maintains healthy hormone levels and contributes to a healthy immune system.

There are two main types of fiber, soluble and insoluble; both support a healthy digestive system. Soluble fiber, found in oats, some mushrooms, legumes, fruits, and vegetables, forms a gel-like substance that can bind to and carry away excess estrogen. Insoluble fiber, found in whole grains, nuts, and seeds, adds bulk to stools, helping move waste through the digestive system, which helps to eliminate excess estrogen.

While healing, I avoided dairy and red meat because I was concerned that the animal's natural hormones and fats might exacerbate endometriosis. I also educated myself about estrogenic foods, which contain compounds called phytoestrogens that can mimic the effects of estrogen in my body. Avoiding them when eating a whole, primarily plant-based diet was challenging, but I did eliminate all soy-based products.

I shifted my diet to around 70 percent raw or lightly steamed produce. I ate only organic and cleaned it well because I discovered it is only considered organic until shipped. Once produce leaves the farm, it may become contaminated. Overseas containers are treated with rodent and insect fumigants and other gases that delay or speed the ripening of the produce. Fumigants can infuse into the products we're eating; these chemicals can wreak havoc on our endocrine system.

In my early twenties, I lived in an apartment that frequently had insects. I had a bottle of chlordane and would saturate cotton balls and place them around the perimeter of my apartment. I later discovered that chlordane is classified as an endocrine disruptor, which can interfere with the normal functioning of hormones, including estrogen. In addition, studies have suggested that chlordane stays in the body for years and can mimic the effects of estrogen. As a result, I've always wondered if chlordane contributed to my developing endometriosis or lupus. I wondered, could the fumigants used in our food supply and manufacturing contribute to immune illnesses?

Being aware of the toxins used during growing, harvesting, processing, transportation, and storage helped me to make healthier choices. Another discovery I made was that aside from wheat and peanuts potentially having mycotoxin contamination that can weaken my immune system, some flours are treated with chlorine dioxide, benzoyl peroxide, or potassium bromate—all things I didn't want in my body. I also discovered that wheat is estrogenic, and it's not on the candida diet. All signs pointed to eliminating it from my diet. Still, I had a family to feed, and I loved to eat bread occasionally. So, I researched and found that using sourdough starter and grinding organic wheat berries into flour was the healthiest alternative to store-bought. I'm not a fan of restrictive diets. I believe we heal because we listen to our body's signals. Listening to my body and eating in moderation is what I did to heal. I didn't fixate on any one diet.

With any autoimmune disease, vigilance in protecting the body from hosting other parasites is vital. A weakened body is a magnet for opportunists. To reduce the possibility of fungus or parasitic infection from food sources, I cleaned store-bought hard-skinned fruits and vegetables well by first rinsing them, then rubbing them with sea salt, letting the salt sit on the skin for five to ten minutes, then using a scrub brush as I rinsed the salt off, air-dried the produce, then stored it in the refrigerator. Likewise, I'd soak leafy greens and berries in a 50/50 saltwater solution with a tablespoon or two of apple cider vinegar, lemon juice, or hydrogen peroxide for fifteen minutes, then rinse and store it in the refrigerator. I recently came across a study (https://pubmed.ncbi.nlm.nih.gov/29067814/) suggesting that a solution of baking soda and water can effectively remove pesticide residues in approximately fifteen minutes. None of these effectively eliminate the chemicals these plants absorb while growing, but they do help to remove the sprayed residue on the outside of them.

Eventually, I learned that ozone could degrade pesticide residue on produce and effectively kill some mold and bacteria. So, I ozonated the water that I soaked my produce in. Purchasing local organic produce is the best choice. If you live in the north as I do, I suggest you harvest and freeze as much local organic produce as possible to get you through the winter. Mind you, my discoveries were back in the early '90s, well before there was much talk about gut dysbiosis or probiotics!

Eliminating Candida Through Diet

Postoperatively, I would experience joint pains, severe abdominal pain, and a whitish tongue for weeks following each surgery; my research led me to discover that an overgrowth of candida was causing these symptoms. So, another goal after this surgery was to eliminate foods that fed candida.

Unfortunately, each hospitalization presented a relapse of ill health and candidiasis caused by the stress of surgery and the bouts of antibiotics given during surgery. Following the surgery with Dr. Reich, I still developed a yeast-coated white tongue, but the historical post-surgery abdominal pain was significantly reduced. I was making progress toward healing but still struggled with candida. It took me years to tweak my diet and heal my gut.

I remember telling a friend that I craved drinking a beer or eating something sweet every day around 4:00 p.m. Once I healed my gut, those cravings went away. I swear that the candida was looking to be fed every afternoon!

In medical jargon, a recurrence of lupus symptoms is called a "flare." I was convinced that these flares were triggered by the stress of successive surgeries or the ensuing usage of antibiotics, anesthesia, and surgical and postoperative medications, which intoxicated and overwhelmed my already delicate body and further suppressed my immune response. This often led to overgrowth of candida and an intoxicated bowel and body. It was cyclical and a common post-surgical consequence that took me years to understand and months to recover from after each operation.

The more progress I made, the more questions arose. For example, could a candida-induced suppressed immune system have contributed to developing an autoimmune disease? Could I cure lupus if I rebalanced the candida in my colon? Was lupus caused by a leaky gut, where food proteins leaked into my bloodstream, causing an immune response every time I ate?

At some points, I could not eat anything I enjoyed without feeling ill effects immediately. I went to a fabulous doctor, Dr. Beasley, who was well-known for diagnosing food allergies and offering vitamin IV therapy. According to testing, I came up allergic to 80 percent of what I ate, and I was malnourished. I was diagnosed with a leaky gut. He said that the nutrients I was eating weren't being absorbed and nourishing my body. I was sensitive to everything I loved to eat. When the body struggles with a leaky gut, it's hyper-sensitive and can trigger an immune response to foods eaten. Dr. Beasley's office could help diagnose and provide nutrition via my veins, but they didn't know the underlying cause or how to fix it. "Leaky gut" was a new term back in the early '90s. I was on my own.

There are many layers to healing, including determining which diet is best and figuring out where to start. The more research I studied, the more confusing healing was; there was conflicting information, and I needed to know which foods to eat and which to avoid. Healing a leaky gut and maintaining healthy gut flora was essential to healing. This process takes patience, faith, and dedication to honoring and listening to our bodies. The term "leaky gut" is ambiguous, and many theories, supplements, and programs are available online today to support and guide healing. Unfortunately, little was documented on healing a leaky gut when I was diagnosed.

Healing my leaky gut was a delicate balance of trial and error and listening to my body, but I believe that the enzyme I was taking for adhesions was monumental in sealing the deal. I stuck to a healthy diet, reduced toxins, maintained a health-promoting home environment, exercised, was optimistic, meditated, etc. I was doing all the right things and was feeling fabulous for months. I was convinced I'd healed myself of everything! Then I'd go out for dinner or to a party and eat and drink whatever was served. Shortly after that, I'd begin experiencing stomach upset, fatigue, joint pain, and headaches lasting for days and sometimes weeks.

It was easy to forget what suffering felt like when I had felt great for so long. After these setbacks, I was pessimistic, thinking I'd never heal myself fully and that I'd have to limit my enjoyment of food and drink for the rest of my life if I wanted to feel good.

Biofilms, the Appendix, and the Gut

Those thoughts lasted a hot moment, and then I returned to researching and trial and error. I wondered, if I truly had my leaky gut and candida under control, then why was my body reacting so severely to the foods I ate at a weekend party? At some point, I came across a Klaire Labs article about biofilm and how candida, bacteria, and viruses work together in the colon to create a protective barrier that shields them from the host's immune system and medications designed to eradicate them. In other words, biofilm is the microorganism's survival mechanism to protect itself from the effects of drugs and the body's immune system. Unfortunately, these biofilms can negatively alter the gut microbiome, impacting digestion, nutrient absorption, and immune function.

Intriguingly, the Klaire Labs article discussed the same enzyme I had been taking to dissolve adhesions and prevent their recurrence. The enzyme, diet, and lifestyle changes had been effective for endometriosis pain, so I had stopped taking the enzyme. The article mentioned that the enzyme effectively dissolves biofilms, allowing the host's immune system or medications to do their job.

I knew my symptoms were triggered by what I ate, but I couldn't understand why my body reacted harshly to one or two meals. Once again, more questions. Could it be that once I went back to eating a less healthy diet, the candida in my colon triggered the biofilm to release its contents to overpopulate my colon? Were my symptoms solely from an overpopulation of candida, or did zonulin, the protein it produces, damage my intestinal lining again, leading me back to a leaky gut? Could the enzyme dissolve the biofilm, letting me finally win this cyclical battle? I had to test it out.

I adhered to my healthy eating 100 percent, practiced mindfulness, positivity, and gratitude, meditated, exercised, grounded in nature, focused on self-care, hydrated, reduced toxic burden, supplemented my diet with probiotics first thing each morning, and took the enzyme each night before I went to bed, hoping it would end the vicious cycle. I loved my body up, and it worked! Over time, my pain subsided, I felt energized, my low-grade fever normalized, my joint pains were gone, my bowels were happy, and stomach pain and endometriosis were a thing of the past.

While researching, I read some interesting information that might factor into why I struggled with candida and leaky gut for so long. When I had my first surgery at age 15 to remove an ovarian cyst, the surgeon also decided to remove my appendix. In the early 2000s, an immunologist at Duke University proposed that the appendix plays a role in the immune system by providing a "safe house" for beneficial gut bacteria. Beneficial gut bacteria play a role in regulating the growth of candida and protecting against infection. Perhaps some of us who struggle to balance our gut microbiota struggle because we don't have an appendix.

Healing is a deliberate, communicative, and disciplined mind-body practice. I was acutely in tune with my body, listening, feeling, and lovingly responding. Sometimes I'd become tired of the strictness, thought it wasn't helping, abandoned the diet for a day or more, and paid dearly. Then I'd get right back up, dust myself off, and forge ahead with compassion, faith, and forgiveness. I was continually assessing and pivoting if need be.

Chapter 8

EMUNCTORIES: THE IMMUNE SYSTEM'S DREAM TEAM

After getting my leaky gut and candida under control, I shifted my focus to strengthening my immune system. I delved into understanding what can stress the immune system and how to nurture it back to health. I learned through gemmotherapy studies that proper functioning of all emunctories is vital for maintaining health and preventing disease. Emunctories refer to the organs or systems that eliminate waste products and toxins. These include the lymphatic system, liver, kidneys, intestines, lungs, and skin.

> **The more consciousness you bring into the body,**
> **the stronger the immune system becomes. It is as if every**
> **cell awakens and rejoices. The body loves your attention.**
> **It is also a potent form of self-healing.**
> **—ECKHART TOLLE**

Understanding The River of Life

The lymphatic system is the body's understated dynamo. It protects us from invading bacteria, viruses, and other microscopic invaders, and destroys cancer cells. It filters our blood while nourishing our cells.

For the lymphatic system to function efficiently, it must flow unimpeded. Our lymphatic system relies upon breath and movement of the body to move lymphatic fluid throughout the body; unlike the heart, it doesn't have a pump to circulate its fluid.

When the lymphatic fluid is stagnant or restricted, toxins can build up in the body, leading to negative symptoms such as headaches, migrating aches and pains, fatigue, and more. Envision a fish tank whose filtration system isn't functioning efficiently. It's toxic, and the fish become sick and die unless we clean the tank. The same is true for our lymphatic system.

Our lymphatic system is made up of the following parts:

- *Lymph nodes* are part of our body's defense system. These small, bean-shaped structures can be found in various areas of the body and help to fight infection, filter lymphatic fluid, and protect us from illness.

- The *spleen* plays an integral role in maintaining a healthy body. It filters blood and removes old or damaged red blood cells. It also helps produce white blood cells that fight infection.

- The *thymus* is a small gland in the chest that plays a crucial role in developing the immune system. It produces and matures T-cells, a white blood cell type that helps fight infection. The thymus is most active during childhood and early adolescence and begins to shrink and become less active after puberty.

- *Bone marrow* plays an important role in producing red blood cells, white blood cells, and platelets. It also contains lymphocytes, a type of white blood cell involved in the immune system's fight against infection.

- *Tonsils and adenoids* are located at the back of the throat and act as a first line of defense, trapping and eliminating harmful bacteria and viruses that enter the body through the mouth and nose. These organs can help protect us from serious illnesses and reduce our risk of infection.

- *Peyer's patches* are clusters of lymphoid tissue located in the small intestine. They help to protect the body against harmful bacteria and other pathogens that enter the digestive system.

When our lymphatic system becomes overloaded with toxins, it doesn't function efficiently, which can result in various unpleasant symptoms such as:

- Digestive issues such as bloating, constipation, or diarrhea
- Swollen and painful lymph nodes
- Fatigue
- Skin issues, such as acne, rashes, hives, or dry skin
- Joint pain and stiffness
- Headaches or migraines
- Allergies and sensitivities
- Poor immune function

Our lifestyle choices can have a major impact on our lymphatic system and overall health. For example, physical inactivity, toxins in our food and water, emotional stress, nutritional deficiencies, tight clothing, antiperspirants, vaccinations, medications, alcohol consumption, excess caffeine, pollutants, and dehydration all stress the lymphatic system.

Tips for a Healthy and Harmonious Body

Lymphatic system

Staying hydrated is my number one tip for supporting your lymphatic system. Drink the cleanest water possible. Begin each day with a large glass of room-temperature water and continue sipping water throughout the day. I invested in a high-quality whole-house water filtration system because I was connected to the public water supply; the chemicals used in the purification process add toxic burdens to the body. We also had high iron concentrations in our water because we were at the end of the water line, so it was important to filter our water. I filled a half-gallon (64 oz.) glass bottle with water each morning and aimed to finish at least one bottle daily. I also used a timer on my watch to remind me to drink hourly.

Daily exercise helps to move lymphatic fluid. Check my chapter on movement and exercise for ways to move your body and minimize pain. The lymphatic system relies on muscle action to pump lymphatic fluid throughout the body. Tight clothing and wired bras constrict the flow of lymphatic fluid, supporting stagnation and toxicity.

Chronic stress is a big one. It can impair lymphatic function. When your body is under stress, the sympathetic nervous system is activated, releasing stress hormones such as cortisol and adrenaline. These hormones cause constriction of blood and lymphatic vessels, reducing the flow of lymphatic fluid and impairing lymphatic drainage. In addition, stress can weaken the immune system, making it harder for the body to fight infections and diseases. Finally, prolonged stress causes muscle tension and poor posture, which can pressure the lymphatic vessels and obstruct the flow of lymphatic fluid. Incorporate stress management techniques such as meditation, yoga, or deep breathing exercises into your daily routine to reduce the effects of stress.

Dry brushing is a technique that involves brushing the skin with a soft-bristled brush to stimulate lymphatic flow and remove dead skin cells. A luffa sponge is my favorite option for dry brushing and skin cleansing. They're natural and effective at exfoliating while gently stimulating the lymphatic system. To learn more, look on YouTube for a demonstration video published by a certified lymphatic drainage massage specialist.

Incorporating healthy habits into a daily routine can help support optimal immune function. Check out my chapters on movement and supplements to discover other ways I kept my lymphatic system happy and healthy.

Liver

Our livers are incredible, with their ability to perform a wide range of essential functions that help us stay healthy. The liver plays a role in metabolism and cholesterol synthesis, regulates hormones, detoxifies the blood, stores glycogen and vitamins, manufactures proteins, and supports the immune system. The liver supports our immune system by producing proteins that help destroy invading microbes. In addition, it produces cytokines, signaling molecules that regulate the immune response, and it manufactures immunoglobulins or antibodies responsible for recognizing and neutralizing foreign substances in the body. It also makes proteins that can help reduce inflammation and promote tissue repair. What a powerhouse organ!

Protecting and nourishing my liver was a priority, and one of the reasons I decided to avoid taking medication. Many medications can cause liver damage. I loved my liver (and still do!) and wanted it to live a long, healthy life. I was never a fan of alcohol but indulged when out with my friends; I knew it wasn't nourishing my liver, so I eliminated alcohol when healing. I also focused on reducing toxins and chemicals by stopping the use of plastics in food and drink storage. Supporting my body's natural detoxification, I stayed hydrated and drank from glass bottles and ceramic mugs instead of Styrofoam and chemically treated paper cups. As mentioned, I installed a whole-house water filtration system to reduce chemical exposure.

My diet was primarily plant-based whole food, but there were times when my family wanted processed foods, so I read every ingredient before putting anything into my cart and would find a way to make it myself if the prepared version was laden with toxins. One of my favorite little books to bring shopping was *Food Additives: A Shopper's Guide to What's Safe & What's Not* by Christine Hoza Farlow, D.C.

I frequently visited the Environmental Working Group's website to learn which products to avoid. Today, they offer research and reviews on everything related to staying healthy. Their mission is stated as: "To empower you with breakthrough research to make informed choices and live a healthy life in a healthy environment." I focused on becoming aware of everything that came in contact with my body, from body care to laundry soap, and either made my own or purchased nontoxic products (you can learn more about this in the chapter about environmental toxins). The more I could reduce toxic exposure, the happier my liver and I would be. Nurturing my liver during my lupus healing journey was a pivotal part of regaining my health, and it remains a cornerstone of my ongoing commitment to well-being.

Urinary system

When I was first diagnosed with lupus, lupus nephritis was a big concern because I had a long history of kidney stones and urinary tract infections (UTIs). I wanted to learn what causes infections and burdens kidneys to keep them healthy. To minimize damage to my liver and kidneys, I decided early on that I wouldn't take traditional medications or over-the-counter non-steroidal anti-inflammatories (NSAIDs). I felt worse when taking them, so it didn't surprise me when I researched them and discovered that many of the medications could do more harm than good.

Knowing which medications can cause kidney inflammation and damage is essential; there are many, such as certain antibiotics, immunosuppressants, NSAIDs, and antivirals. Educate yourself and research a medication to make an educated decision for your body. If it isn't curing something, question it. If it is, question it. If a new symptom arises, discuss it with your physician, hydrate, move your body, and tap into your soul to ask for guidance. Doctors want to help you alleviate symptoms, but time is often the best cure. If you are there at the doctor's office, they expect that you are there because you want them to solve your problem; and generally, the solution is in the form of a pharmaceutical or treatment, i.e., charting your symptoms and noting what makes them worse or better. Be patient and loving to your body; give it time to heal. Additionally, I requested alternative diagnostic tests if a CT or MRI scan with contrast was ordered. Contrast agents can injure the kidneys.

To support urinary health, I kept myself hydrated with at least half a gallon of water daily, and drank homemade fruit and veggie electrolyte broth, raw juices, and herbal and cornsilk teas. It's important to note that drinking only water can lead to electrolyte imbalances that can cause symptoms such as dizziness, nausea, and muscle cramps. Dehydration, conversely, can make us feel agitated, weak, tired, headachy, and thirsty and cause muscle cramps. In addition, dehydration can lead to a rapid heartbeat, confusion, and fainting. Some days when I was underhydrated, I'd feel overly tired and have a slight headache by early afternoon; this was my warning sign that I forgot to drink enough that day. So I'd add a pinch of sea salt and a squeeze of lemon to my water, drink it, and perk right up. I set an hourly timer to prevent dehydration and remind myself to drink.

Drinking water is essential for proper hydration and kidney health, but it should not be the only focus. Maintaining a balanced and varied diet that includes a variety of nutrient-rich whole foods, such as fruits, vegetables, whole grains, lean protein, and healthy fats, is essential for keeping the body happy and healthy. Our diet plays a significant role in our health, and processed, cooked, and animal-based foods contribute to increased acid in the body, which leads to inflammation.

Our body works hard to maintain pH balance; if it didn't, we'd die. This work is done primarily by our kidneys. Eating a healthy percentage of raw foods can support our kidneys and lessen the acidity burden, whereas processed, cooked, fatty foods increase that burden. Simply stated, an acidic body is an inflamed body. So, what's a healthy percentage? There is no one-size-fits-all answer to what is a healthy ratio of raw food to cooked food. The ideal balance largely depends on your commitment to healing yourself, your preferences, and your overall health status. Easing into change by experimenting with raw food and listening to your body is my best advice; whether it's 5 percent, 10 percent, or 80 percent raw is up to your mind and body.

While navigating my healing, I first focused on learning what was healthier than what I was eating. I had been anorexic and bulimic for a few of my teenage and young adult years, so I had much to learn. I studied numerous dietary theories and took from each what resonated with my body while using whole food as my foundation.

I discovered that a whole-food, primarily plant-based diet worked best for me. While I loved party foods, sweet, salty, crunchy snacks, and fast food, I knew they wouldn't support my healing.

Healing myself was a full-time, disciplined commitment. I committed to loving my body beyond any love it had ever experienced; by doing so, I enhanced my mind-body communication, an intuition and respect that propelled my healing.

I experimented with my diet, listening to my body for clues and honoring them. At different times during the healing decade, I craved or had an upset digestive system from various foods, and when I did, I observed those messages by eating what it craved and eliminating what upset it. The more intently I listened and honored, the faster I healed.

Hypertension (high blood pressure) can damage your kidneys, so monitoring your blood pressure regularly and taking steps to keep it under control is essential. Blood pressure monitors are available for home use and can be purchased over the counter inexpensively. High blood sugar can also damage the kidneys, especially if you have diabetes. So, managing your blood sugar levels is important as well.

To prevent recurrent bladder infections, I had to educate myself on what caused them. Dehydration can contribute to a bladder infection by reducing the frequency and volume of urination, leading to an increased risk of bacterial growth in the urinary tract. Impeccable hygiene is the number one priority. Tampons harbor bacteria that contribute to vaginal and urinary tract infections. Strings from the tampons can introduce E. coli bacteria into the urinary tract. If you wear them, change them frequently, and to protect the urinary tract from colon bacteria, it's important to wipe from front to back 100 percent of the time. Sexual activity can increase infections; both partners should shower before intercourse, and women should visit the bathroom and urinate to flush bacteria out of the urethra immediately following relations. Change sweaty workout clothing and wet bathing suits promptly. Bacteria and yeast love warm, moist environments, and tight, damp clothing supports their growth, as does wearing tight underwear to sleep at night. Wear loose cotton pajama shorts or nothing at all. These simple preventative steps can help eliminate UTI suffering and keep your immune system healthy.

The urinary system, like a silent guardian, plays a crucial role in bolstering our body's immune defenses. Picture it as the keeper of the body's internal harmony, responsible for maintaining vital balances. When it's in good health, it stands ready to shield us from invaders. The immune system thrives when the urinary system is in sync. Think of it as a dynamic partnership—the kidneys, like vigilant sentinels, filtering and purifying, and the immune system, an army of defenders. Together, they ensure our body remains resilient and ready to combat threats.

Intestines

This part of my digestive system was stressed, too, because I had had numerous operative procedures that manually manipulated my colon. In addition, I was burdened with endometrial implants that caused adhesions that attached my colon to other organs in my body. (In Chapter 7 I shared my plan to eliminate adhesions and candida, which supported my intestines in healing.)

Our intestines play a crucial role in maintaining a healthy body. They help to ensure that we can absorb the necessary nutrients from our food and eliminate waste products from our bodies. If you struggle with intestinal distress, make it a priority to lean in and figure out what is causing it and correct the underlying cause. Don't settle for "it's a result of having lupus" or take a prescription. Instead, take the time to explore the underlying cause and lovingly correct it. Only you have the answers.

Lungs

Like the kidneys, the lungs are responsible for maintaining homeostasis. Homeostasis is the body's ability to maintain stable internal conditions despite changes in the external environment. The lungs play a critical role in maintaining homeostasis by regulating the concentration of gases in the body, particularly oxygen and carbon dioxide. Through the gas exchange, the lungs help maintain the body's acid-base balance by eliminating excess carbon dioxide, preventing acidosis, and ensuring optimal oxygen levels in the blood. Maintaining healthy lung function is crucial for maintaining homeostasis and overall health.

While studying yoga, I discovered that deep diaphragmatic breathing could increase my lung capacity and improve circulation, enhancing my body's natural detoxification process. Proper breathing techniques help to increase oxygen levels in the body, promote relaxation, and stimulate the parasympathetic nervous system, which is responsible for the "rest and digest" response. When we breathe deeply and rhythmically, we take in more oxygen, which can help stimulate the production of white blood cells, boost the immune system, and aid in eliminating toxins from the body.

Deep diaphragmatic breathing can be done anytime. With regular practice, this exercise can help to improve your well-being. Set an intention that's aligned with your healing, then:

- Sit or lie down in a comfortable position. You can place one hand on your chest and the other on your belly to feel the movement of your breath. Close your eyes and focus on the sensations you feel.

- Take a few deep breaths to relax your body and clear your mind.

- Inhale slowly and deeply through your nose, allowing your belly to expand as you draw air into your lungs.

- Exhale slowly through your mouth, letting your belly fall as you release the air from your lungs.

- Focus on the sensation of your breath as it moves in and out of your body. You can count to four as you inhale, hold your breath for a count of four, then exhale for a count of four, then hold this exhale for a count of four, then repeat this cycle for several breaths.

If you're not feeling up to exercising, breathwork is a lifesaver.

Skin

Some scientific evidence suggests that the skin may play a role in eliminating certain toxins from the body. One way is through the process of sweating. Sweat is a mixture of water and electrolytes produced by the sweat glands in the skin; it also contains small amounts of toxins.

Another way our skin may play a role in detoxification is through sebum excretion. Sebum is an oily substance produced by our skin's sebaceous glands. It helps lubricate the skin and hair and traps certain toxins.

I decided to focus on nourishing and protecting my skin; it's always protecting and looking out for me. As mentioned, I love the sun, and instead of slathering on a chemically processed sunblock, I primarily made my own, using coconut oil and iodine. I made body scrubs from olive oil, sea salt, and sugar, and body butters using shea butter, coconut, jojoba, mango seed oil, and honey combinations. I created bug repellants using essential oils and made my own haircare, laundry, and kitchen products. It was a lot of work, so I eventually sourced them using the Environmental Working Group's research. You can learn which products are safest at www. ewg.org/skindeep.

When we take the time to show love and care for our organs, we create a positive and nurturing environment that supports their healthy function. This, in turn, enables them to perform optimally and efficiently, contributing to our healing and overall well-being. My relentless, obsessive desire to live and heal supported my cure. I would not be alive today had I not done what I did for myself, by myself. I hope my experience inspires you and reminds you that we are all capable of great things and that you should never give up on yourself, no matter how challenging things may seem. Keep asking questions, keep learning, and keep trying new things. Your resilience knows no bounds, so always persevere, no matter the obstacles you encounter.

Chapter 9

MY HEALING
REMEDIES

Much of my healing journey was about *feeling* better. I learned to tune in to my body's signals and lovingly find ways to soothe it. Healing begins with self-awareness and taking care of your body's needs. Quick fixes may seem tempting, but they may only worsen the situation. In this chapter, I provide a concise reference to supplements and holistic remedies that have played a vital role in my journey toward self-healing. Let my experiences inspire you to research further, encouraging you to explore new methods and approaches to support your health and well-being.

Home remedies and supplements have gained popularity, but their effectiveness is often based on anecdotal evidence rather than scientific proof. Approach cautiously. Please consult a healthcare professional beforehand to ensure they are safe and appropriate for your circumstances.

I experimented with various remedies to alleviate symptoms

and boost my immune system during my self-healing journey. I tracked my body's response, noting any side effects or benefits, and I encourage you to do the same. I discovered that relying solely on supplements and natural remedies was not enough, and listening to my body and responding with loving care was crucial.

The following list of supplements and remedies is based on my extensive research and experience using them. My overall focus was reducing the inflammatory burden on my body, because an inflamed body struggles to heal itself.

Enhancing Digestion Naturally

Digestive enzymes

When I started my healing journey, I felt fatigued after meals, even though I ate nutrient-dense foods. It was like my body was working overtime to digest what I had just eaten. So, I experimented with supplements to see if they would help me feel better. After trying different options, I found that taking a digestive enzyme with meals high in fats or proteins made a difference. I no longer felt sluggish and exhausted after eating.

HCL/Betaine

Until I fully healed my gut, I supplemented cooked meals with betaine to support stomach acid formation—low levels of stomach acid support leaky gut and autoimmune disorders. Stomach acid is necessary for proper digestion and absorption of nutrients, as well as maintaining a healthy gut environment. Also, candida overgrowth leads to an imbalance of gut bacteria, which can contribute to the development of small intestinal bacterial overgrowth (SIBO). SIBO can interfere with stomach acid production by disrupting the balance of bacteria in the gut and altering the digestive process. My solution to break this cycle was to take betaine at the start of a cooked meal and digestive enzymes with meals high in fat and protein.

Lemon, sea salt, and ginger

As I continued to heal my gut, I replaced my use of betaine and digestive enzymes with a delicious and effective digestive aid—a blend of lemon, sea salt, and ginger. This powerful trio works together to support the natural production of digestive enzymes.

Ginger's antimicrobial properties curb the growth of harmful gut bacteria. At the same time, sea salt supports the production of hydrochloric acid, and lemon's alkalizing effects reduce acidity levels, promoting better gut health and reducing the likelihood of acid reflux.

This easy-to-make digestive tonic is a versatile addition to any meal, complementing a range of dishes such as fish, chicken, vegetables, or salad. Simply combine 4 tablespoons of freshly squeezed lemon juice, 1 teaspoon of sea salt, and 1 teaspoon of freshly grated ginger. Mix, allow to marinate for a few hours, then add a teaspoon to your meal and enjoy the benefits of this nourishing blend.

 ## The Healing Power of Fermented Foods

Fermentation produces beneficial bacteria that create compounds like short-chain fatty acids and probiotics, known to strengthen the immune system and improve gut health. These foods also reduce inflammation and enhance the absorption of essential vitamins and minerals, making them a great addition to my diet.

Here are several of my favorite healthy ferments:

Kimchi is a delicious fermented dish that combines vegetables like napa cabbage, radishes, and scallions with flavorful spices such as garlic, ginger, and chili flakes. The fermentation process produces lactic acid and beneficial probiotics that aid digestion and absorption of nutrients. Kimchi is also high in fiber and anti-inflammatory spices, which can help regulate digestion and reduce gut inflammation.

Sauerkraut is chopped cabbage fermented with salt and its juices. This process creates beneficial bacteria that produce lactic acid, which gives the sauerkraut its tangy flavor. People from many cultures enjoy sauerkraut as a condiment or side dish. It's packed with soluble and insoluble fibers and helpful bacteria that promote good digestion.

Studies have shown that fermented foods like kimchi and sauerkraut are great for gut health because they contain helpful bacteria and are rich in fiber, vitamins, and minerals. However, the specific strains of bacteria and their concentrations may vary, leading to slightly different benefits. For example, kimchi usually has *Lactobacillus plantarum*, which can help with digestion and inflammation in the gut, joints, and skin. Sauerkraut, on the other hand, has more *Lactobacillus brevis* and *Pediococcus pentosaceus*, which can improve digestion and immunity while reducing inflammation throughout the body.

If you're not a fan of sour foods, buy a small jar of kimchi from your local store and add a teaspoon to your plate. Eat it raw as a condiment, or mix it into your salad. Compared to sauerkraut, kimchi is milder on the sour scale but can be spicy. Read the ingredients before purchasing. You can easily make both kimchi and sauerkraut at home. There are many recipes online; experiment until you find one you love. Sandor Ellix Katz is one of my favorite fermentation gurus; he's written some fantastic cookbooks.

Apple cider vinegar (ACV): There's a lot of documentation that touts ACV's healing properties. I've found it helpful in reducing indigestion and nighttime reflux. It contains acetic acid that stimulates gastrin production, which regulates stomach acid. ACV also activates digestive enzymes that break down food and can lower the stomach's pH, making it easier to activate pepsin, which breaks down protein. And on top of that, the acidity of ACV can also kill harmful bacteria and pathogens in the stomach.

I'd drink one tablespoon in a quarter-cup of warm water an hour after a meal to reduce nighttime indigestion. Another way is to use ACV in cooking, such as adding it to salad dressings or marinades. Some people prefer to take ACV supplements in the form of capsules. It's important to note that undiluted ACV is too harsh for the throat and digestive system, so diluting it before consumption is recommended.

The Power of Sea Salt

Another side effect of my lupus was idiopathic orthostatic hypotension, which caused sudden drops in blood pressure when standing up. The symptoms were severe, and I would have to squat and hold onto something until the blackness faded before standing up again. Unfortunately, there wasn't anything the medical community could do to help me because they couldn't find a cause.

In addition, chronic stress had elevated my cortisol levels. Cortisol is a hormone released in response to chronic stress, and high levels over time can weaken the immune system and increase the risk of chronic disease. Reducing stress while fighting for your life is difficult, but I knew I had to take steps to bring balance back to my cortisol levels with regular exercise, meditation practice, and better sleep.

While learning how to correct these imbalances, I found anecdotal information suggesting a solution called solé might help reverse hypotension and support adrenal gland health due to its numerous natural minerals and trace elements. Solé is a concentrated saltwater solution made from sea salt, not table salt. Table salt and sea salt are both types of salt, but they have some key differences in composition and processing. Table salt is mined from underground salt deposits and is heavily processed to remove minerals. It is typically comprised of 97-99% sodium chloride and is often fortified with iodine. On the other hand, sea salt is produced through seawater's evaporation and contains small amounts of minerals and trace elements that are not present in table salt. Such trace minerals are essential for good health.

I felt rejuvenated by adding a teaspoon of solé *solution* to my morning water. Not only did it alleviate my orthostatic hypotension, but it also contributed to the normalization of my cortisol levels and effortless bowel movements. Consult your doctor before adding solé to your daily routine.

Create a batch of solé by adding 1 teaspoon of sea salt to a cup of filtered water. Store the mixture in a covered glass jar and let it sit until the salt crystals dissolve. Then dilute one teaspoon of the concentrated solé in an 8-ounce glass of water and drink it first thing in the morning on an empty stomach. While solé is purported to offer various health benefits, scientific evidence remains limited.

Bone Broth and Gelatin

Bone broth is a liquid produced by simmering animal bones for an extended period. This broth is reputed to assist in healing a leaky gut, so I incorporated it into my wellness routine. The broth is rich in beneficial nutrients such as collagen and gelatin, which help strengthen the gut lining and reduce inflammation. Additionally, it is a good source of vital minerals including calcium, magnesium, and phosphorus, all of which support a healthy gut.

I obtained beef bones from an organic farmer, washed them before rubbing them with sea salt, and roasted them in the oven for 45 minutes. I then simmered the bones in water for 12 to 15 hours to make a flavorful broth. Once cooled, I strained the broth using a wire colander and stored it in eight-ounce glass jars, which I froze for later use. To consume, I thaw the broth in the refrigerator overnight, heat it on the stovetop the next day, then sip it directly or incorporate it into a soup with raw vegetables such as parsley, mushrooms, and scallions, or even add an egg for a hearty lunch. Chicken or fish bones can also be used to make broth, but strain the stock meticulously to eliminate any small bones. Intriguingly, a Google search for broth recipes yielded over 28 million results.

Gelatin was an inexpensive multifaceted lifesaver! As someone with lupus, I struggled with brittle nails with bumpy vertical lines. I was determined to find a solution; then, I discovered the benefits of gelatin, a great source of collagen for the strength and elasticity of hair, nails, and skin.

Not only did gelatin support my hair and nail health, but it also helped to improve my gut health. The amino acids in gelatin, such as glutamine, proline, and glycine, played a crucial role in repairing and regenerating my intestinal lining, improving digestion and nutrient absorption.

I would typically mix two teaspoons of gelatin in a cup of hot water until dissolved, squeeze in half a lemon, and sip it warm on an empty stomach. Gelatin's water-absorbing properties helped to keep my digestive tract hydrated and promoted healthy bowel movements. The glycine content in gelatin also helped to reduce inflammation in my gut, while the proline content supported the growth of beneficial gut bacteria.

After two months of consistently supplementing with gelatin, I noticed that my hair and nails became thicker, and the ridges in my nails disappeared. Overall, gelatin proved an affordable and multifaceted solution that supported my hair, nail, and gut health!

 ## Castor Oil Packs

Castor oil packs have been used for centuries as a natural remedy for various health issues. They are typically used to promote healing, reduce inflammation, and improve circulation in the body. For example, I used castor oil packs to prevent constipation, minimize adhesions, and alleviate joint pain.

I made castor packs by saturating 20" x 4" flannel strips in organic castor oil. I laid down a large plastic bag before applying the strips to avoid staining my sheets. Then I placed the strips horizontally across my abdomen from just under breasts to just above the pubic bone. After covering the packs with another plastic bag and a towel, I placed a hot water bottle or heating pad on top of them for 30-45 minutes. When I had joint inflammation, I wrapped the affected area with castor oil strips and used plastic wrap to hold them in place. Then I wrapped the heating pad around for added relief. The packs provided excellent pain relief and helped ease and sometimes prevent post-surgical pain and constipation.

 ## Pain-Relieving Epsom

I found some relief by taking Epsom salt baths to ease my muscle and joint pain. The magnesium and sulfate in Epsom salt are absorbed through the skin, aiding in muscle relaxation, inflammation reduction, and joint stiffness and pain relief.

To make an Epsom bath, fill the bathtub with warm water. Add one to two cups of Epsom salt to the water and mix until dissolved. Then soak in the bath for at least twenty minutes.

 ## Cooling Showers

As I embarked on my lupus journey, I stumbled upon an unexpected realization: hot showers were zapping my energy levels! Despite their soothing effect on my achy joints, the steamy heat left me feeling drained and exhausted. But I wasn't about to give up on my precious shower time, so I devised a crafty solution.

Halfway through my usual hot shower routine, I'd close the drain and let the warm water rise up to my ankles, creating a cozy pool of warmth for my feet. Then, I'd gradually lower the temperature of the shower water while keeping my feet warm. The refreshing cool water left me feeling invigorated and ready to tackle the day ahead.

I should mention that my lupus journey didn't involve Raynaud's syndrome, which can be triggered by cold water. So, if you're dealing with this condition, you might want to steer clear of the chilly showers!

 ## Restoring Balance for Candida Recovery

What follows is a brief explanation of my understanding of candida's role in the body and what happens when it's out of balance.

Candida is a normal part of the human body's microbiome, the collection of microorganisms that live on and in our bodies. Candida is a type of yeast generally found in small amounts in various parts of the body, such as the mouth, throat, gut, and vagina. It helps to break down food particles and extract nutrients, and it can also help to prevent harmful bacteria from overgrowing in the gut. Candida can stimulate the immune system and promote the production of antibodies, which can help to protect the body against infections. It helps to maintain the natural pH balance of the vagina and prevent the overgrowth of harmful bacteria. Some studies have suggested that candida can help promote wound healing by stimulating the growth of new cells and preventing infections.

In healthy individuals with a balanced microbiome, the presence of candida is not usually a cause for concern. However, when there is an overgrowth of candida, it can lead to infections, leaky gut, and other health concerns. This overgrowth may occur due to a weakened immune system, antibiotic or corticosteroid use, chronic stress, hormonal changes, or a diet high in sugar and refined carbohydrates. Conditions caused by candida overgrowth include oral thrush, vaginal yeast infections, systemic candidiasis, and immune system dysfunction.

I developed an overgrowth of candida. In the early stages of my diagnosis, the physicians thought I had Lyme Disease and administered strong antibiotics intravenously; I was also given high doses of prednisone to reduce painful inflammation. Before this, I was being treated for PCOD, or polycystic ovary disease, and had several surgeries to remove ovarian cysts and endometriosis. Candida overgrowth became my body's way of life, making it challenging to heal.

Candida overgrowth wreaks havoc on our bodies in several ways:

- *Disrupting the gut microbiota:* Candida overgrowth disrupts the balance of beneficial bacteria in the gut, which play a critical role in regulating our immune system. When the gut microbiota is imbalanced, it can lead to chronic inflammation and impair the immune system's ability to fight infections.

- *Producing toxins:* Candida produces toxins such as acetalde-hyde and ethanol, which can damage our immune cells and impair their function. These toxins can increase inflammation and oxidative stress in the body, further weakening our immune system. An accumulation of acetaldehyde in the body can affect the motility of the colon and cause fatigue, brain fog, and digestive problems.

- *Affecting neurotransmitters:* An overgrowth of candida in the gut may affect the production and balance of gut neurotransmitters, such as serotonin, dopamine, and gamma-aminobutyric acid (GABA). Candida overgrowth can lead to inflammation and damage to the intestinal lining, which can affect the production of neurotransmitters. For example, some studies have shown that candida overgrowth can cause a decrease in serotonin levels in the gut, leading to symptoms such as abdominal pain, constipation, and diarrhea. Serotonin is an important neurotransmitter that regulates many functions in the gut, including motility, secretion, and sensation. Candida overgrowth may also affect the balance of other neurotransmitters, such as dopamine and GABA, essential in regulating mood, appetite, and other aspects of brain function.

- *Modulating immune cell activity:* Candida can adjust the activity of immune cells, such as T-cells, by altering their cytokine production and immune function. Cytokines are a group of signaling molecules produced by our immune cells and other types of cells in response to infection, injury, or inflammation. The balance between pro- and anti-inflammatory cytokines is vital for maintaining proper immune function and preventing excessive inflammation. In lupus, some T-cells can activate and produce cytokines that promote inflammation and tissue damage.

- *Damaging intestinal cells:* Candida overgrowth can produce enzymes that interfere with digestion. For example, Candida albicans can produce an enzyme called phospholipase, which can break down phospholipids in cell membranes, damaging intestinal cells and causing intestinal permeability, also known as "leaky gut." This damage to the intestinal lining can increase gut permeability, allowing larger molecules such as undigested food particles, toxins, and bacteria to pass through the intestinal wall and into the bloodstream. This can trigger an immune response, leading to inflammation and other health problems.

Because of all these negative effects, addressing candida overgrowth to support the immune system and prevent reinfections was a top priority.

 ## The Key Supplements on My Healing Journey

Monolaurin is a natural compound found in coconut oil and human breast milk. Monolaurin has been shown to have several potential health benefits, including protecting against infections, supporting digestion, improving skin health and preventing acne, and improving overall heart health by reducing cholesterol levels. I took monolaurin to reduce inflammation and prevent or reduce the overgrowth of candida following my surgeries.

Colostrum is a nutrient-rich substance produced by mammals in the first few days after giving birth. Colostrum contains various immune-boosting compounds and growth factors that can help support gut health and repair the intestinal lining.

Some healing benefits of colostrum include:

- *Boosting immunity:* Colostrum contains high levels of immunoglobulins, which are antibodies that help to protect against infections. These antibodies can help boost the immune system and protect against various pathogens.

- *Fighting infections:* In addition to immunoglobulins, colostrum also contains other immune-boosting compounds such as lactoferrin, cytokines, and growth factors, which can help to fight infections and reduce inflammation in the body.

- *Promoting tissue repair:* Colostrum contains growth factors such as insulin-like growth factor 1 (IGF-1), which can help promote tissue repair and regeneration. Colostrum may be particularly beneficial for healing leaky gut syndrome.

- *Supporting gut health:* Colostrum contains prebiotics and probiotics that can help to support the growth of beneficial bacteria in the gut. This can help to support gut health and boost immunity; our gut is an essential part of our immune system.

I drank organic bovine colostrum to boost my immune system and support gut health. If I couldn't find it fresh or frozen, I'd choose a product derived from grass-fed cows that was minimally processed to preserve immune factors, had been third-party tested for quality and purity, and contained no additives or fillers.

Glutamic acid encourages the growth of beneficial gut bacteria, such as bifidobacteria and lactobacilli, which help to maintain a healthy gut microbiome. It also helps to strengthen the gut lining by improving tight junctions between gut cells, reducing the risk of the leaky gut syndrome. I supplemented with glutamic acid while healing leaky gut. The presence of bifidobacteria and lactobacilli in the microbiome is associated with a healthy gut, reduced inflammation, improved gut barrier function, and the growth of beneficial bacteria. Conversely, decreased bifidobacteria and lactobacilli levels are associated with candida overgrowth.

Deglycyrrhizinated licorice root (DGL) is licorice root with the compound glycyrrhizin removed, which can cause side effects such as high blood pressure and low potassium levels in some individuals. DGL is commonly used as a natural remedy for various digestive issues and may have healing benefits for the gut. Here are some potential healing benefits of DGL:

- *Soothes the digestive tract:* DGL can help to soothe the lining of the digestive tract and reduce inflammation. It may benefit individuals with acid reflux, gastritis, and inflammatory bowel disease.

- *Supports gut health:* DGL can help to support gut health by promoting the growth of beneficial bacteria in the gut and reducing the growth of harmful bacteria. It also helps to protect the gut lining and promote tissue repair.

- *Promotes mucus production:* DGL can help promote mucus production in the digestive tract, which can help protect the gut lining from damage and irritation.

- *Supports healthy cortisol levels:* DGL may help support healthy cortisol levels, which can benefit individuals with adrenal fatigue and other stress-related conditions.

- *Reduces pain and discomfort:* DGL may help to reduce pain and discomfort associated with digestive issues, such as acid reflux and stomach ulcers.

I found DGL soothing and a welcome addition to my healing toolbox. Candida overgrowth produces toxins that can irritate the digestive tract. This inflammation can interfere with the production of stomach acid, which is essential for breaking down food and absorbing nutrients. So when I had acid reflux, instead of taking over-the-counter antacids, I found that DGL alleviated my symptoms and supported my healing.

Oregano oil has been shown to have antifungal properties due to its high content of a compound called carvacrol. Carvacrol is effective against a variety of fungi, including candida.

As with my experiences, speaking with your healthcare provider before using oregano oil is essential. Oregano oil can interfere with the absorption and effectiveness of certain medications. It may also increase the risk of side effects or adverse reactions when combined with certain drugs. In addition, oregano oil is highly concentrated and can irritate the digestive system if taken in large amounts or without proper dilution.

Here are some ways I use edible oregano oil: (It is important to use a high-quality oil labeled for internal use.)

- *Diluted in water:* Add a couple of drops of oregano oil in a glass of water.

- *Mixed with food:* I added oregano oil to salad dressings, marinades, sauces, oil sprays, and dips.

- *Capsules:* Edible oregano oil is available in capsule form, making it easier to consume and to control dosage.

- *Oil pulling:* I used oregano oil in oil pulling, which involves swishing a small amount of oil around in the mouth for a few minutes before spitting it out. It's an ancient Ayurvedic practice believed to improve overall health by removing toxins from the body, reducing inflammation, and boosting the immune system. I'd add a couple of drops to a tablespoon of coconut oil, swish for five minutes, and then spit it out.

Serrapeptase: This enzyme was originally discovered in the intestines of silkworms, where it helps to dissolve the tough cocoon and allows the silkworm to emerge as a moth. However, the serrapeptase enzyme used in dietary supplements is produced through microbial fermentation using bacteria. Serrapeptase has been shown to have anti-inflammatory and pain-relieving properties and may also help break down harmful biofilms.

As mentioned in Chapter 7, I took serrapeptase (from World Nutrition in my case) to dissolve adhesions and later learned about its benefits against candida biofilm. I took serrapeptase on an empty stomach at bedtime. Then, in the morning, I would take the probiotics on an empty stomach.

Probiotics: Supplementation with probiotics is beneficial when dealing with candida overgrowth because it helps restore healthy gut bacteria balance. Probiotics are live microorganisms similar to the beneficial bacteria naturally found in the gut. When taken as a supplement, probiotics can help to repopulate the gut with beneficial bacteria, which can help to improve digestive health and support the immune system. I healed from lupus over thirty years ago; very few probiotics were available back then. The one I used was called Primal Defense. I'd mix a scoop in a glass of water each morning and drink it before breakfast.

Flora Sambu Guard syrup: When training to become a nurse, I was concerned about exposure to illnesses and looked for a supplement to support my immune system. Flora Sambu Guard incorporates two botanical ingredients—elderberry and echinacea—which have a longstanding history of being utilized for immune support. It kept me healthy!

Vitamins and other traditional supplements: When I saw Dr. Beasley, and he diagnosed me with leaky gut, he prescribed the following supplements (purchased in my case from Metagenics), which I took three to four times a week for several years: magnesium, potassium, Omega-3 fatty acids, vitamin D, and the Multigenics multivitamin.

Iodine: I supplemented with iodine because I had learned that a deficiency might contribute to cystic conditions in the body, and I had breast, ovarian, and liver cysts. I took a couple of drops of Lugol's iodine in my water a couple of times a week.

NAC: N-acetylcysteine is a precursor to glutathione, a powerful antioxidant that supports the body's ability to remove toxins and support liver function. It also helps to reduce inflammation in the body. I took NAC to prevent severe Herxheimer reactions while managing candida and detoxifying my body.

Metagenics Mycotaki: This supplement is a concentrated mushroom formula with seven nourishing mushroom extracts traditionally used to support the immune system. I took it for extra immune support during stressful times.

Rescue Remedy: A natural remedy made from flower essences, Rescue Remedy was developed by Dr. Edward Bach. It helps reduce stress and anxiety, promotes relaxation, improves sleep quality, and supports emotional well-being. I'd take this remedy when I was anxious or stressed, and it would provide rapid natural relief without side effects.

Natural Vitality Calm: Sometimes lupus affected my muscles, sleep, and stress levels, and it was challenging to get a good night's sleep. This magnesium supplement was a lifesaver. I took the original formula in a glass of water each night before bed and would sleep comfortably for hours and wake up refreshed.

Boiron Quietude: This homeopathic remedy temporarily relieves sleeplessness without causing grogginess or dependency. This remedy proved miraculous on nights when I experienced difficulty falling back asleep after waking up in the middle of the night. I'd take one or two tablets under my tongue, and by the time they'd finished melting, I'd be back in dreamland.

Amrita Deep Rest Essential Oil: People with lupus who have poor sleep quality have a higher risk of experiencing pain, fatigue, depression, and anxiety. Lack of sleep can weaken the immune system, which is already compromised. So, I made sure that I had a good night's sleep. I'd put a dab of this delightful essential oil on my shoulders and pillow to prepare for rest. It's a great essential oil for unwinding after a long day.

Cortisol Manager: During my ongoing studies to maintain health after lupus, I learned about Cortisol Manager from Integrative Therapeutics, a dietary supplement containing a blend of herbs and nutrients that support healthy cortisol levels and relaxation in times of stress. I rely on this supplement to calm me during prolonged stress or when I struggle to get a good night's sleep.

Cortisol Manager is commonly used to support individuals with stress-related conditions such as anxiety, insomnia, and adrenal fatigue. I discovered Cortisol Manager after I healed from lupus while looking for something to help me with insomnia. Cortisol

Manager helps me fall asleep and get a good night's sleep. I take it as needed. Good sleep is essential to staying healthy. As a result, I wake each morning feeling well-rested and refreshed.

Banyan Botanicals Healthy Hair: Another remedy I used for a few years was Healthy Hair. At times, my hair was falling out by the handful. Hair loss was exacerbated by anesthesia; each time I had surgery, I'd experience massive hair thinning for months following. This Ayurvedic supplement works. Over time, my hair grew back thicker than it had ever been.

Bee pollen: I suffered from seasonal allergies and discovered that bee pollen could help alleviate my symptoms. I became a beekeeper and collected pollen from the bees in early spring, storing it in the refrigerator for the following season. In anticipation of spring allergies, I started a month-long regimen. Each morning, I'd mix a half teaspoon of bee pollen into a spoonful of either honey or almond butter, savoring the spoonful as a proactive shield against the upcoming itchy eyes and runny nose.

My goal was desensitization—exposing my body to pre-seasonal pollen in small amounts to reduce reactivity, akin to traditional allergy shots. Though I can't claim immediate results, I've been free from spring allergies for almost thirty years.

Keep track of when you're most sensitive to pollen, seek local beekeepers selling bee pollen around that time, and store the pollen in the refrigerator to begin consumption before next year's allergy season. Note that pollen consumption, especially in unprocessed forms, carries potential risks, including allergic reactions, foodborne illnesses, and drug interactions. Allergies can vary significantly in severity and triggers, making it important to recognize that what works for one person may not be suitable for another.

Even small amounts of pollen could worsen symptoms for some individuals. Therefore, it is strongly advised to consult with your healthcare provider before incorporating pollen into your routine.

GABA and California poppy: Throughout my ten-year healing journey, two supplements became invaluable companions: GABA and California poppy. GABA, or gamma-aminobutyric acid, emerged as a steadfast ally. As a natural chemical produced by the brain, it acts as an anti-anxiety neurotransmitter. Recognizing that chronic stress depletes GABA levels, I decided to incorporate daily GABA supplementation into my routine. It required patience, a virtue I often lacked, but after several months of consistency, I discovered a remarkable shift. I experienced a heightened sense of relaxation and found it easier to maintain optimism. GABA played a pivotal role in alleviating both my physical pain and anxiety by countering the detrimental effects of stress.

Alongside GABA, I found solace in the gentle embrace of the California poppy plant. This extraordinary plant holds within its essence natural compounds that possess remarkable properties. They soothe anxiety, reduce stress, and provide relief from pain. To this day, I consciously choose to reach for my California poppy tincture when acute pain strikes, bypassing over-the-counter pain relievers. Its rapid and potent effectiveness is a reliable natural remedy.

From Shamans to Backyard Harvests

I enjoy using God's gifts to heal myself. Many of those gifts were right in my backyard. When I traveled, I sought local shamans, traditional healers, and herbalists to learn about their region's wild edibles and medicinal plants.

I mention the plants I used to pique your interest and prompt your research. I researched some plants for months before deciding to ingest them. Be cautious, and listen to your body. Each plant has many healing properties, but also contraindications. Pick one that interests you and research it. Before harvesting and using any plant, take time to learn about its properties, and consult an ethnobotanist or herbalist and learn about proper harvesting, preparations, health benefits, toxicities, and contraindications. Plants are medicine, so please check with your doctor before using them.

Less inflammation meant less pain, so I mainly focused on plants that offered anti-inflammatory properties, but I fell in love with the healing properties of some other plants along my journey. I will share some of them with you below. I typically ingested these as teas, both hot and cold. Sometimes I'd add dried organic apple, pineapple skins, lemon, lime, orange peels, cinnamon sticks, nutmeg, cardamom, cayenne, dehydrated strawberry, or mint to enhance the flavor.

White pine needles: This was my favorite winter hike tea. When I'd locate a white pine tree, I'd collect fresh needles to brew tea when I returned home. These needles contain vitamin C and other antioxidants that help to support my immune system and reduce inflammation. To make a delightful immune-boosting white pine needle tea, rinse and finely chop one tablespoon of fresh needles. Steep them in a cup of hot water for 5-15 minutes, covered. Strain the tea and enjoy it hot, adding honey for sweetness or lemon for a zesty twist. Learn about your pine trees! This will help you identify which varieties are safe to use for tea-making.

Dandelion roots: I love all parts of the dandelion plant, but the roots make the best tea. It tastes a little bitter, almost like coffee. This is my go-to drink instead of caffeinated tea or coffee. It's delicious and has powerful immune-boosting and anti-inflammatory properties. Dandelion root tea is believed to support liver health by promoting the flow of bile, which helps remove toxins from the liver. It may also help protect the liver from damage caused by free radicals.

Mugwort: Most people call it an invasive weed here in the American Northeast. However, science loves to study this plant for cancer, where it's been found to induce apoptosis (cell death) in cancer cells. It's also been found to have potent antifungal and anti-inflammatory effects, inhibiting the production of pro-inflammatory cytokines. So I decided to drink it to support my efforts of controlling candida overgrowth. I harvest the plant from spring to late fall; the root and leaves are dried and used in tea.

Elderberry: I love this delicate and beautiful flowering plant. Raw elderberries are toxic and must be cooked before ingesting. I drank elderberry tea to support my immune system and reduce seasonal allergies.

Lotus Root: This root has been used in traditional Chinese medicine for thousands of years to promote kidney health. It's a natural diuretic that helps to increase urine output, flushing out toxins and waste products from the kidneys.

Juanilama: I was introduced to juanilama tea by an indigenous woman in Costa Rica. This tea soothes the digestive tract, reduces inflammation, and boosts the immune system.

Blackberry leaf: The tannins in blackberry leaf tea are believed to have anti-inflammatory properties. I harvested the leaves throughout the summer, air-dried them, then made a cold brew tea that included some of the berries.

Rosa rugosa: This beautifully fragrant rose shrub makes a delicious vitamin C tea. In the early fall, after all of the roses have bloomed, I harvest the rosehips, allow them to air dry, and then add them to my other dry tea blends. Vitamin C is known to boost the immune system.

Cornsilk: This delicate silk is a lifesaver. Anyone who's had a bladder infection knows the frustrating pain. I've had several kidney stones and bladder infections, and this tea has reliably prevented me from needing antibiotics or anti-inflammatory bladder medications. I'd always have a small bag of cornsilk in my freezer.

Graviola: Also known as soursop, it is a bitter herb often used in traditional medicine as a bitter tonic. Bitters are plant-based substances believed to have anti-inflammatory and antioxidant properties. I learned about this powerfully healing plant during a visit to Costa Rica, where the fruit, leaves, and bark are used in natural remedies. I drank tea from the leaves to support my digestive health.

Exploring Gemmotherapy and Plant Stem Cells

Gemmotherapy is a form of phytotherapy that uses extracts from the buds, shoots, and young roots of plants to enhance detoxification and promote healing. For safe and effective use of gemmotherapy, it's important to seek guidance from a certified gemmotherapist.

I used the following extracts to support detoxification and reduce inflammation:

- *Betula Pendula/Birch bud extract:* Birch bud extract has diuretic properties, which can help eliminate toxins and waste products through the kidneys and urinary system.

- *Ribes Nigrum/Blackcurrant bud extract:* Blackcurrant bud extract supports the liver and promotes the elimination of toxins through the bile. It is also thought to have a diuretic effect, which can help eliminate toxins and waste products through the kidneys and urinary system.

- *Common hornbeam bud extract:* Common hornbeam bud extract is believed to have a stimulating effect on the lymphatic system, which can help to increase the elimination of toxins and waste products.

- *Juniper bud extract:* Juniper bud extract has a diuretic and detoxifying effect on the kidneys and a cleansing effect on the digestive system.

- *Rosemary bud extract:* Rosemary bud extract is believed to stimulate the liver and promote the elimination of toxins through the bile.

- *Zea mays rootlet extract:* Zea mays is derived from the rootlets of corn and is indicated for kidney and bladder inflammations.

I am eager to share an astounding experience that serves as compelling evidence of the remarkable effectiveness of gemmotherapy. More than fifteen years ago, a close relative was diagnosed with Tourette's syndrome, burdened with uncontrollable tics like lip licking, eye blinking, and throat grunting for an extended period. However, the transformative power of gemmotherapy became evident when they started taking daily doses of Ficus carica and Tilia tomentosa extracts. Miraculously, within just one week, the tics vanished completely and never resurfaced. This undeniable connection between gemmotherapy and healing beautifully illustrates the potency of nature's wonders.

Chapter 10

ENVIRONMENT: REDUCE, REDUCE, REDUCE!

The possibilities for healing are vast and endless. During my healing journey, I realized the importance of thorough exploration. To truly leave no stone unturned, I embraced the mantra of "trust your intuition." If a thought or idea came to mind, I allowed myself to explore it further. I understood the significance of conducting diligent research to determine whether it held the potential for my healing. Being open to new possibilities and actively seeking knowledge left no avenue unexplored in my pursuit of healing.

Knowledge about environmental health detriments is vital for improving and preserving overall health. While these harmful effects may not be visible, they exist in the air, water, food, soil, dust, and our household and personal products. Therefore, being aware of your surroundings and minimizing exposure to these toxins is vital.

Minimizing exposure to environmental hazards can boost our well-being and help us attain optimal health. Consider beginning this journey by reevaluating your current body care and household products and exploring healthier alternatives. Question their potential side effects, and stay open to discovering new options. By being open-minded, you may find solutions that better align with your health goals.

To help with this effort, the Environmental Working Group website provides valuable information on safe personal care and cleaning products that can help you reduce your exposure to household toxins. Use their site as a guide to prompt further research. Manufacturers may change their formulations, so stay vigilant about reading labels.

Below I share some of my discoveries, hoping to inspire your exploration. With a fervent determination to regain my health and live a long, fulfilling life, I embarked on a relentless path toward healthier options.

At first, I approached some of the research and treatments skeptically, but I knew I had nothing to lose; doctors had given my life a rapidly approaching expiration date. And indeed, my efforts paid off. However, it's important to note that I'm not a scientist or doctor; please find what resonates with you on your unique healing journey and continue to discuss your decisions with your doctor.

In the following sections, I summarize some valuable ways that I explored to support my healing. I hope that they serve as inspiration for you and encourage further research on your part!

Identifying Environmental Hazards: Air, Water, Food, and Beyond

Air

Clean air is a fundamental necessity for our overall well-being. Our lungs are the gateway to our bodies, and the air we breathe impacts our health. Polluted air can contain harmful particles, including dust, pollen, mold spores, pet dander, and even toxins from vehicle emissions and industrial pollutants. Breathing in these contaminants burdens our immune system and can lead to various health issues, from respiratory problems and allergies to more severe conditions like asthma and cardiovascular disease.

By prioritizing clean air, we reduce our risk of illness, improve respiratory function, boost energy levels, support healing, and enhance our overall quality of life. To improve indoor air quality, consider the following steps:

- Identify and minimize potential sources of indoor air pollution like dust, pet dander, tobacco smoke, cleaning products, mold, and volatile organic compounds (VOCs)—organic chemicals that easily evaporate, contributing to indoor air pollution. They come from various sources such as building materials, furniture, carpets, paints, solvents, and cleaning products. Identifying VOCs can be challenging, but you can read product labels, review Material Safety Data Sheets (MSDS), pay attention to strong odors from new products, research product information, and look for low-VOC or zero-VOC alternatives. They're often listed as eco-friendly or non-toxic. VOCs can have short-term and long-term health effects, including respiratory issues and organ damage. Consult an indoor air quality professional for guidance and testing if concerned about VOC exposure.

- Regularly clean and vacuum to remove dust, pet hair, and particles from surfaces and carpets. Use a vacuum cleaner with a HEPA filter for utmost effectiveness.

- Ensure proper ventilation by opening windows, using exhaust fans in kitchens and bathrooms, and promoting airflow to reduce indoor pollutant concentration.

- Use portable air purifiers with HEPA filters, especially in frequently occupied rooms.

- Check and change the air filters in your HVAC system regularly. This prevents the recirculation of polluted air throughout your home or office. Follow the manufacturer's recommendations for the frequency of filter replacement. Have your air ducts professionally cleaned to remove accumulated dust, debris, and potential contaminants.

- In addition to changing the air filters in your HVAC system, it is important to change the air filters in your car. The air filters in your vehicle help ensure you are not inhaling pollutants while driving. Refer to your car's manufacturer guidelines for the recommended frequency of air filter replacement.

Improving indoor air quality is an ongoing process. Regular maintenance, cleaning, ventilation, and filtration create a healthier and cleaner environment to support your healing.

Water

Clean water is vital to our overall well-being and is essential for numerous physiological processes; it helps regulate body temperature, aids digestion and nutrient absorption, lubricates joints, flushes out waste and toxins, and supports the proper functioning of our organs and systems. When we consume and bathe in clean, filtered water, we provide our body with the pure hydration it needs to function optimally, promoting healing, vitality, and overall health. Clean water is not just a necessity but a fundamental element for our body's well-being.

Drink and bathe in clean, filtered water to reduce exposure to toxins and support your body's healing. Installing a reliable water filtration system, like activated carbon filters or reverse osmosis systems, removes impurities effectively. Countertop or under-sink filters are practical choices for a cost-effective water filtration solution. Additionally, installing a shower head with a built-in filter can help reduce chlorine, heavy metals, and impurities in bathing water. Regular maintenance and filter replacements ensure optimal filtration performance. Also, stay informed about local water quality through reports and guidance from health authorities for necessary precautions.

Before installing a whole-house water filtration system, I would feel exhausted after each shower. My research revealed that this exhaustion was likely caused by the disinfection chemicals in the water. When the immune system is suppressed, we can become more sensitive to substances that wouldn't usually cause a reaction for us. The off-gassing of these disinfection chemicals during a hot shower may have played a role in my exhaustion.

For a convenient and safe hydration option while on the go, consider filling a couple of glass bottles with filtered water from your home and bringing them along with you.

Food

The famous quote "Let food be thy medicine and medicine be thy food," often attributed to Hippocrates, carries even greater significance today. With the modern food supply being modified and laden with toxins, artificial additives, and pesticides, it becomes essential to prioritize clean, organic food for our well-being. Hippocrates' wisdom underscores the importance of consuming natural, unprocessed foods that can nourish and heal our bodies. We minimize exposure to harmful chemicals and promote healing by choosing organic options. Making conscious choices to prioritize clean, organic food is a powerful way to embrace food's healing potential and support our overall health and vitality.

Although organic food is typically more expensive, there are strategies to make it more affordable. Shopping at local farmers' markets or joining a community-supported agriculture (CSA) program can provide reasonably priced fresh organic produce. Planning meals, buying in bulk, and growing herbs, vegetables, or fruits can also help cut costs. Consider purchasing organic staples in larger quantities from bulk bins or online, and prioritize seasonal produce in meal planning. By implementing these approaches, it's possible to incorporate clean, organic food into your diet without over-stretching your budget.

Fields

EMF, short for electromagnetic field, is a form of energy in our surroundings, originating from power lines, cellphones, electronic devices, and the planet. Although not typically considered toxins, EMF has the potential to impact our health, and further research is necessary to safeguard our well-being.

An article published in *Environmental Pollution* titled "Immunotoxicity of radiofrequency radiation" discusses recent research that suggests radiofrequency radiation (RFR) could be a new environmental pollutant that may harm our immune system. Scientists have examined how RFR affects specific immune cells that help protect our body from illness. They found that RFR can cause changes in the way our immune cells work. Scientists recommend conducting more studies to test different types of RFR and see how they might harm our immune system. It is essential to understand this because exposure to EMFs is pervasive.

Despite being invisible, EMFs can pose potential health risks, making it essential to minimize exposure. To reduce these risks, consider maintaining a safe distance from sources like cell phones, Wi-Fi routers, and power lines. Limit exposure time by taking breaks and turning off devices at night. EMF shielding products such as phone cases, shielding fabric, laptop shields, and grounding sheets can provide additional protection. Opting for hardwired connections like Ethernet cables and wired headphones can also help minimize exposure to EMFs. By implementing these strategies, you can take proactive steps to reduce potential health risks associated with EMF exposure.

Geopathic stress

This is the belief that certain environmental factors, such as electromagnetic fields, underground water veins, fault lines, mineral deposits, and human-made disturbances, can disrupt our health. While there is limited scientific evidence to support this belief, I preferred to take a cautious approach and proactively address potential risks in line with my focus on well-being.

The theories explaining geopathic stress vary. Some suggest that the earth's natural electromagnetic field can become distorted or intensified, leading to imbalances in the body's electrical systems when exposed over time. Others argue that underground water veins or geological disturbances emit harmful energies that can disrupt the body's natural processes. Prolonged exposure to these geopathic stress factors might weaken the immune system, disrupt cellular function, disturb sleep patterns, and potentially contribute to chronic conditions such as fatigue, headaches, and general discomfort.

During my healing journey, I decided to investigate the potential impact of these fields on my health. So, using a TriField EMF meter, I measured magnetic fields in areas where I spent the most time; for example, my bed, office chair, and kitchen. If the meter reading was high in these areas, I moved the furniture to an area with a lower reading. Higher meter readings may indicate elevated magnetic field levels that could pose health or safety concerns and weaken my body.

We can't eliminate it, but we can reduce it. Understanding how invisible external forces might affect the body's electrical balance is complex and continually evolving. Further research is needed to fully comprehend the mechanisms involved and their potential implications for human health. In the meantime, it is best to be aware and take steps to mitigate exposure.

The *Schumann resonances*, often called the Earth's "heartbeat," is a natural electromagnetic resonance in the Earth's atmosphere and is believed to offer several health benefits. It arises from the interaction of lightning discharges with the Earth's surface. The fundamental mode, resonating at approximately 7.83 Hz, represents the dominant frequency within the Schumann resonance range. Exposure to the Schumann resonances promotes relaxation, reduces stress, improves sleep quality, enhances cognitive function, and supports overall well-being. It is seen as a harmonious connection to the Earth's energetic rhythm, fostering balance and vitality.

To experience the positive effects of the Schumann resonances, you can spend time outside in nature in parks, forests, or by the water, where there's less manufactured electrical interference. In addition, walking barefoot or sitting or lying on the ground can help you connect with the Earth's natural electromagnetic field.

Radiation reduction

Every day we encounter various types of radiation, including electromagnetic radiation like radio waves, microwaves, visible light, and X-rays. Among these, ionizing radiation such as X-rays and gamma rays possess enough energy to affect the atoms in our cells and harm their DNA. Thankfully, our cells have an impressive ability to repair this damage using their built-in mechanisms. However, if the repair process goes awry, it can lead to cell death or even cancer development. While our bodies possess defense mechanisms against DNA damage caused by ionizing radiation, limiting excessive exposure to minimize potential health risks is crucial.

I included antioxidants like N-acetylcysteine (NAC), alpha-lipoic acid (ALA), vitamins C and E, and beta-carotene in my diet to reduce my risk. While natural supplements cannot guarantee complete protection against ionizing radiation, scientific research suggests that antioxidants can help combat the oxidative stress caused by radiation exposure. I also took the initiative to question the necessity and potential risks of specific medical procedures, such as X-rays and CT scans. For example, I chose to forgo mammography and embrace MRI as a safer alternative. By opting for MRI, which avoids using low-dose X-rays, I aimed to minimize my risk of radiation exposure. Exploring and discussing options with healthcare professionals is essential to make informed decisions aligning with our health goals.

Despite my lupus diagnosis, I deliberately decided to find a middle ground regarding sun exposure to aid my healing process. Instead of avoiding sunlight altogether, I chose to moderate my exposure. I took essential precautions like using natural sunscreen, wearing protective clothing and sunglasses, and seeking shade during the sun's peak hours. In addition, regularly checking the UV index enabled me to evaluate the intensity of UV radiation, aiming for a lower UV rating to minimize my exposure and adjust my activities accordingly. By striking a balance, I ensured that I considered both the positive effects and potential risks of sunlight. Taking proactive steps and making informed decisions contribute to our overall well-being.

Mold

Mold is insidious as it grows in hidden areas, develops slowly, and can negatively affect us. In addition, its ability to thrive in concealed spaces makes detection difficult until it has spread extensively. As a result, the health effects of mold may not be immediately recognized as related to exposure. It's essential to be aware of mold in your home and take steps to reduce its impact on your health.

Mold can affect the immune, respiratory, and nervous systems. It can cause allergies and inflammation, and weaken our ability to fight off illnesses. In addition, mold exposure can lead to various neurological symptoms, including headaches, dizziness, difficulty concentrating, memory problems, fatigue, and mood or behavioral changes. It can be associated with conditions like tremors, neuropathy, and cognitive impairments in severe cases.

Mold typically grows in areas of homes where moisture is present. Common locations include bathrooms, kitchens, basements, attics, crawlspaces, laundry rooms, windowsills, and areas affected by water damage. These areas often have higher humidity levels, poor ventilation, or water leaks, providing an ideal environment for mold to thrive. Regular inspection and addressing moisture issues are crucial in preventing mold growth.

During my thirties, I noticed that I developed a constant cough, but it only occurred when I was inside my office. I had a suspicion that something in the room was the cause of my cough, even though I couldn't visually pinpoint the source. It was discovered that we had mold growth underneath the carpet. To tackle the issue, they removed the carpet and meticulously cleaned the underlayment using a mixture of bleach and water. Next, they set up fans and heaters to dry the area thoroughly. To ensure no trace of mold remained, an ozone machine was used to eliminate any lingering mold spores. The result? My cough symptoms vanished, and I could finally breathe easier. If you ever face a mold problem, I highly recommend contacting a professional mold remediation expert—they can make a world of difference.

Mold is a stealthy problem with significant health impacts. Proactive measures such as regular inspections, prompt moisture issue addressing, and appropriate remediation are crucial for minimizing its presence. By being vigilant and taking the necessary steps, you will reduce the risks of mold exposure.

Nurturing a Healthier Home and Body

During my healing journey, I took the initiative to make some of my products at home. Also, I made informed purchases with the guidance provided by the Environmental Working Group. Visit their website to make informed decisions on personal care products. They provide recommendations for products and offer the EWG VERIFIED™ seal, which signifies products that meet their rigorous standards for safety and transparency. You can easily find trusted products that align with your preferences for safer and healthier choices.

House cleaning

Some house cleaning products can be toxic, depending on the specific product and its ingredients. Many household cleaners contain chemicals such as ammonia, bleach, and sodium hydroxide, which can be harmful if inhaled. These chemicals can cause skin irritation and other health problems; certain cleaning products release VOCs into the air, leading to respiratory problems and other health issues. When the body is immunocompromised, these chemicals can further burden it, so finding healthier alternatives is best.

Here are a few healthy alternatives I use; remember to test them on a small area before using them.

- *Baking soda* is a gentle cleaner and deodorizer, suitable for scrubbing surfaces and absorbing odors. It's a versatile and practical product that simplifies cleaning tasks around the house. When mixed with water, it's an all-purpose cleaner for countertops, sinks, and stovetops. It acts as a deodorizer, eliminating unpleasant odors in the refrigerator, pantries, carpets, and upholstery. I refresh my carpet by combining a few drops of lavender essential oil with two cups of baking soda. I sprinkle this mixture onto the carpet, let it sit for an hour, and vacuum it. Baking soda can be combined with vinegar to clear clogged drains, sprinkled in the dishwasher to freshen, or added in the laundry to brighten whites. With its versatility and effectiveness, baking soda is a healthy option for household chores.

- *Castile soap* is a vegetable-based, biodegradable, and practical all-purpose product. I use it for hand soap, dishwashing and laundry detergent, plant spray to deter insects, and shampoo. Its wide range of applications makes it a practical and eco-friendly alternative for various cleaning tasks throughout the entire home.

- *Essential oils* such as tea tree, lemon, lavender, and peppermint are my favorite choices for house cleaning due to their antimicrobial properties and pleasant scents. Tea tree oil is effective against bacteria, viruses, and fungi, while lemon oil provides a refreshing and deodorizing effect. Lavender oil offers a calming aroma and is gentle on surfaces, while peppermint oil has an invigorating scent. I add a few drops of essential oil to distilled water in a spray bottle to make a homemade all-purpose cleaning solution. I prefer distilled water because my tap water, although filtered, may still have minerals that may leave a film behind.

- *Hydrogen peroxide* is a non-toxic alternative to bleach. It kills bacteria and viruses and is ideal for disinfecting surfaces. I make a cleaning solution with hydrogen peroxide using equal parts of hydrogen peroxide (3 percent concentration) and water. Then, I store it in a labeled glass spray bottle in the kitchen for sanitizing the table, countertops, sink, and sponges. It works best when sprayed on surfaces then allowed to sit for a couple of minutes before wiping down. Wear gloves when using it, test the solution on a small area before using it on colored surfaces or fabrics, and avoid using it on natural stone.

- *Lemon juice* is a natural cleanser and disinfectant. I dilute it in distilled water in a one-to-one ratio in a spray bottle. Then spray the mixture on a soft cloth and wipe down my wooden furniture, cabinets, and cutting boards.

Laundry

Some laundry detergents may contain chemicals such as phosphates, surfactants, and fragrances that can be harmful to our health and the environment. On the other hand, eco-friendly detergents with gentle, plant-based ingredients are less likely to cause skin irritations. In addition, they are free from toxins commonly found in conventional detergents, such as phosphates, chlorine bleach, optical brighteners, and synthetic fragrances. Avoiding these harmful substances is essential for our health as they can negatively impact our immune system, trigger allergies and skin sensitivities, contribute to respiratory issues, and disrupt hormonal balance.

Removing these chemicals promotes healing and creates a healthier environment for ourselves and others. For example, I make a non-toxic, environmentally friendly laundry soap by combining two cups of washing soda, two cups of baking soda, one cup of citric acid, a half cup of coarse sea salt, and a few drops of lavender essential oil. I mix the ingredients thoroughly and store the mixture in an airtight container. I add three tablespoons of homemade soap to a load of laundry in my washing machine, and my clothes come out clean and smell great!

Dryer sheets and fabric softener

Due to my sensitivity to the chemicals in dryer sheets and fabric softeners, which cause skin irritation and headaches, I decided to explore alternative options. I switched to wool dryer balls and infuse them with a few drops of lavender essential oil. By including these scented balls in my laundry, I achieve a pleasant fragrance and eliminate the discomfort and headaches associated with conventional products.

Dishwashing detergents

Dish soaps can contain toxins and harmful chemicals, which can leave a residue on dishes. After washing, rinse dishes thoroughly with clean water to remove any remaining detergent and minimize the risk of ingesting toxins. Consider switching to natural or eco-friendly detergents free of harsh chemicals. You can make your dish soap products using simple ingredients like baking soda, vinegar, and castile soap.

Body scrub and moisturizer

Create a delightful homemade body scrub by combining one cup of sugar, 1/4 cup of liquid coconut oil, and 10-15 drops of your favorite organic essential oil. Mix well and adjust the ingredients to achieve your desired consistency. I prefer a sugar scrub, but salt can also be used. Next, rub a small amount on dry skin in a circular motion to loosen dry skin cells, then follow up with a warm shower.

Create your own whipped body butter with this simple recipe. Melt one cup of shea butter, 1/2 cup of coconut oil, and 1/4 cup of sweet almond oil in a double boiler. Let it cool for 10-15 minutes, then add 10-15 drops of your favorite essential oil. Place the mixture in the refrigerator for one hour to partially solidify. Use an electric mixer to whip the mixture until light and fluffy, about 5-10 minutes. Transfer to jars and store in a cool place. Apply a small amount to your skin for a luxurious and moisturizing experience.

Perfumes

When I was at my lowest, I had quite a trio of challenges regarding perfumes—persistent headaches, overwhelming fatigue, and frustrating memory loss. Perfumes had a secret vendetta against me because they would unleash these symptoms in full force. The headaches would leave me feeling like my head was in a vise, the fatigue made it a herculean task to get through the day, and the memory lapses turned everyday tasks into a real-life treasure hunt. It was clear that perfumes and I were not a good match. So, I consciously decided to steer clear of them.

Despite the reactions triggered by perfume chemicals, however, I refused to give up on wearing a scent. I discovered the joy of creating my own fragrance using essential oils, nourishing jojoba oil, and vitamin E. It was a game-changer! Amrita became my go-to brand for high-quality organic essential oils, offering divine scents that are pure and natural. With this newfound approach, I could confidently enjoy delightful fragrances without compromising my well-being.

Nail care

Nail polish often contains chemicals like formaldehyde, toluene, and dibutyl phthalate (DBP), which can be absorbed into the body through the skin and bloodstream. These chemicals have been linked to potential health issues, including cancer and reproductive disorders, and may impact the immune system. In addition, acetone, commonly used as a nail polish remover, can adversely affect various organs, making it questionable whether soaking nails in acetone is healthy. However, there is limited research available specifically on the detriments of acetone.

For me, it's essential to exercise caution and consider alternative, less harmful methods for nail polish removal. I apply moisturizing oils like coconut, olive, shea butter, or jojoba to my nails and cuticles. This helps to keep them healthy and shiny. Next, I use a nail buffer to smooth and buff my nails to a polished appearance. It's a quick and easy way to make my nails look their best without subjecting my body to harmful chemicals or treatments that might weaken my immune system.

Oral care

When we experience lupus fatigue, it's easy to overlook the importance of oral care. However, it's essential to understand that maintaining excellent oral hygiene is vital for keeping our bodies healthy and supporting healing. Lupus challenges the immune system, leaving us more susceptible to infections. When we neglect our oral hygiene, it can have significant consequences.

Oral thrush is a common infection in people with compromised immune systems; this happens when the candida fungus in our mouth grows out of control. Factors like prolonged antibiotic use, hormonal changes, dry mouth, or poor oral hygiene can disrupt the balance of candida. Oral thrush can be uncomfortable, causing white patches or lesions on our tongue, inner cheeks, and other mouth areas, making swallowing difficult. If we don't treat it, candida can travel through our bloodstream and cause systemic candidiasis, bringing symptoms like fever, fatigue, digestive issues, skin rashes, joint pain, and organ damage.

Besides oral thrush, the bacteria in our mouth can cause other health problems. The accumulation of bacteria can lead to inflammation, infection, and gum disease. When left unchecked, these bacteria can enter our bloodstream, worsening our illness or leading to new health issues like sinus infections, sepsis, cardiovascular disease, and respiratory infections.

Taking care of my oral health is a personal priority, and I've adopted several practices to maintain a healthy mouth. I brush my teeth several times daily, paying particular attention to my tongue to remove bacteria buildup. Flossing and using a water flosser is essential, ensuring that those hard-to-reach spaces between my teeth stay clean and debris-free. One practice that I've discovered and love is oil pulling. It involves swishing approximately a tablespoon of coconut oil in my mouth for about five minutes. It not only promotes oral hygiene but also leaves my mouth feeling refreshed and revitalized. I add a drop of peppermint or oregano essential oil to my swishing oil. This natural technique has become a favorite part of my routine due to its reported benefits in reducing bacteria and improving gum health. In addition, regular dental checkups play a vital role in detecting potential issues early on.

Early in my healing journey, I made toothpaste using clay, baking soda, sea salt, hydrogen peroxide, and peppermint or clove essential oils. It was a fun experiment! But now, with the convenience of online shopping, I've discovered some fantastic oral care products online. One of my favorites is NaturaRx Dentizyme because it's natural, gentle, effective, and tastes great. Another must-have for me is DrTung's Smart Floss. It's incredible at getting into those tight spots and does an excellent job overall. These products have become staples in my oral care routine, making taking care of my teeth a breeze.

Amalgam fillings

Fortunately, the use of amalgam or mercury fillings has been declining through the years. When it came to concerns about the potential health effects of mercury, I made a proactive decision to have my amalgam fillings removed. These fillings contain mercury, and ongoing debate has been occurring about their impact on overall health. Scientific studies have even suggested a possible connection between mercury exposure and autoimmune conditions. By removing my amalgam fillings, I aimed to decrease mercury exposure and support my immune system.

Nasal care

To support my immune system against excess pollen, bacteria, candida, and viruses, I incorporated daily gargling and nasal rinsing into my routine. Instead of using a neti pot, I made two nasal spray solutions: one composed of sea salt, distilled water, and hydrogen peroxide, and the other containing saline and Lugol's iodine. I sprayed each nostril until the solution trickled down my throat, then expelled it, blew my nose, and repeated with the other spray. With consistent daily use of these practices, I observed a significant reduction in sore throats, sinus infections, and allergic reactions. These habits served as valuable tools in supporting my overall health and immune system.

Cookware

Creating a healthy kitchen environment is about making smart choices regarding your cookware. It's essential to choose materials that are safe for your health. Stainless steel and cast iron are good options because they're sturdy and won't introduce harmful chemicals. Remember that when using cast iron, it's best to be cautious with acidic dishes that cook for a long time, as the acid can interact with the iron and release small amounts of iron into your food.

On the other hand, it's advisable to steer clear of aluminum pots. They have the potential to react with certain foods, which means that a tiny bit of aluminum could end up in your meals. And that's not ideal, because prolonged exposure to high levels of aluminum is linked to health concerns.

Additionally, be cautious about using coated pots classified as nonstick. Over time, when scratched, the coating can flake off and find its way into your food, introducing substances you'd rather avoid. Finally, it's essential to be cautious when using older enamel pots, especially those that were made before regulations were put in place to limit lead content. Some older enamel pots may contain lead-based glazes, including those passed down through generations. With time and use, these glazes can deteriorate, potentially leading to lead leaching into your food. Therefore, it's best to steer clear of enamel pots with unknown origins or those that exhibit signs of wear and deterioration.

The journey to healing from lupus and creating a healthier environment has been transformative. By embracing the mantra of "reduce, reduce, reduce," I opened myself up to endless possibilities for healing. Trusting my intuition, conducting diligent research, and being open to new options led me down a path of exploration that left no stone unturned.

I discovered that our environment plays a crucial role in our overall health. Every aspect has an impact, from the air we breathe to the water we drink, the food we consume, and the electromagnetic fields we encounter. Minimizing exposure to toxins in our surroundings can boost our well-being and support our body's natural healing processes.

My journey to reduce, reduce, and reduce has been marked by persistence, open-mindedness, and a commitment to my health. While I am not a scientist or doctor, I hope my discoveries and experiences inspire your exploration and research. Find what resonates with you on your unique healing journey and continue to discuss your decisions with your healthcare professionals.

By embracing the power of reducing exposure to environmental hazards, we can create a healthier, more supportive environment for our healing and well-being. Remember, the possibilities for healing are vast and endless—trust your intuition, explore new avenues, and let your journey to a healthier environment unfold.

Chapter 11

METAPHYSICAL HEALING & READING SUGGESTIONS

In this chapter we delve into the realm of metaphysical healing, exploring the transformative potential of prayer, visualization, insight, creativity, and divination tools to enhance our overall well-being. Through a journey of spiritual connection and self-discovery, we unlock the incredible power of metaphysical healing to transform our lives.

Metaphysical healing is a holistic approach to wellness that addresses the mind, body, and spirit. It recognizes that we are all interconnected beings, and that our physical and emotional health are influenced by our mental, emotional, and social well-being.

Learn to get in touch with the silence within yourself and know that everything in this life has a purpose. There are no mistakes, no coincidences. All events are blessings given to us to learn from. —ELIZABETH KÜBLER-ROSS

Healing through Introspective Prayer

Prayer is often understood as a means of internal reflection or communicating with the broader universe. Whether viewed through a spiritual lens or not, it can be a way to express feelings, emotions, desires, or gratitude. For many, prayer is about connecting with something outside themselves, seeking solace, comfort, and meaning.

Different cultures and belief systems have their interpretations of prayer. These can range from reciting specific verses to chanting, meditating, silent thinking, and performing particular rituals. The essence of these practices, regardless of form, is seeking understanding, support, and peace.

For me, prayer has been a profound source of personal connection. It allows me to find inner peace, strength, and direction. Especially during turbulent times, it provides stability and a reminder that there's always hope. I've experienced the transformative power of deep introspection and reflection through prayer. It offers a comforting touch, suggesting that positive change and healing are always possible.

Chronic pain or enduring struggles can often shake our foundational beliefs. There might be moments of doubt or feelings of detachment. But I've learned that remaining receptive to the power of introspective reflection is crucial. In such phases, the essence of prayer can be a beacon. At its core, prayer is about reaching out to the vast universe or reaching deep within ourselves.

One approach to this universal prayer is mindfulness and meditation. We can tap into a deep reservoir of peace and understanding by focusing on our breath, being entirely in the moment, or simply expressing gratitude.

Regardless of your background or belief system, embarking on this journey of introspective prayer can be deeply fulfilling. Here are some steps to help you explore this practice:

- *Create a sacred space:* Designate a quiet, peaceful space to feel comfortable and undisturbed during your prayer practice. This space can be a physical area in your home or a place in nature that brings you a sense of serenity and connection.

- *Set an intention:* Before you begin, set a clear intention for your prayer practice. It could be seeking guidance, expressing gratitude, finding inner peace, or sending healing energy to yourself or others. Clarifying your intention helps focus your prayer and gives it purpose.

- *Find a form of expression:* Prayer can take various forms, depending on what feels most authentic. You can express your thoughts and feelings through spoken words, silent contemplation, journaling, visualization, or artistic expression like drawing or painting. Choose a method that resonates with your soul.

- *Cultivate stillness:* Prayer often involves quieting the mind and connecting with a deeper sense of presence. Practice mindfulness or meditation techniques to help calm your thoughts and center yourself before entering into prayer. Deep breathing, focusing on bodily sensations, or repeating a mantra can help create a sense of inner stillness.

- *Speak from the heart:* When you begin your prayer, speak sincerely and genuinely. Share your thoughts, feelings, hopes, and desires. Be open and honest, knowing that you are communicating with a higher power or the universe in a way that feels meaningful to you.

- *Practice gratitude:* Expressing gratitude is a powerful aspect of prayer. Acknowledge and appreciate your life's blessings, experiences, and relationships. Offer thanks for the lessons you've learned and the growth you have experienced, even during challenging times.

- *Seek guidance:* If you seek guidance, pose questions or seek clarity on specific areas of your life. Be open to receiving insights and inspiration during your prayer practice. As you cultivate a deeper connection with your inner wisdom, pay attention to any intuitive messages or signs that may arise.

- *Reflect and integrate:* After your prayer practice, take a few moments to reflect on your experience. Consider any emotions, thoughts, or insights that emerged during your prayer. Integrate the lessons and guidance received into your daily life, applying them to your actions, decisions, and interactions.

Remember, prayer is a personal and evolving practice. Allow yourself the freedom to explore and adapt your approach over time. The most important aspect is cultivating an authentic connection with your inner self, regardless of any specific religious framework.

A Sample Healing Prayer

Dear {Inner Wisdom},

I reach out today with a heart seeking understanding and support. I am navigating the complexities of this chronic condition, and I seek wisdom and guidance as I travel this path of healing.

Please grant me the resilience and strength to face the highs and lows of this journey. Help me discover the most beneficial treatments, therapies, and avenues that foster my physical, emotional, and mental well-being. May I connect with professionals who genuinely understand and can offer the care I need.

I seek clarity about the root causes of my condition and the ways I can address them. Show me habits or patterns that may need change, and guide me toward practices that nourish every part of my being, creating balance and vitality.

As I confront the challenges and limitations of this situation, help me find acceptance and calm even during trying moments. May I always remember that healing is a step-by-step process, and every day brings its own triumphs.

May I be surrounded by understanding and supportive individuals—whether family, friends, or healthcare experts—who stand by me and provide solace. Their presence is a constant reminder that I'm not alone on this journey.

Above all, I release my anxieties and concerns, trusting in the process. May I see the lessons and growth opportunities this condition brings, allowing it to shape me into a more understanding and resilient person.

I am thankful for the support and guidance I feel, knowing that there is a force guiding me toward better health and balance. I appreciate this connection and the encouragement it brings.

With love and gratitude,

[Your Name]

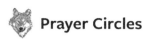 **Prayer Circles**

Invite your loved ones to form a healing circle of prayer on your behalf. Collective prayer possesses extraordinary healing potential, offering a profound source of support, hope, and transformation.

A powerful connection emerges when individuals unite with a shared intention in collective reflection. Participants' combined focus and intent amplify the healing desire, generating a potent field of positive energy. This communal belief in the strength of collective intention, the power of the universe, and human resilience creates a strong resonance that can overcome challenges. It paves the way for unexpected positive outcomes and profound transformations.

 The Transformative Power of Visualization

In the face of life-limiting or chronic illness diagnoses, it's natural for a wave of negative thoughts and emotions to surge, including fear, anxiety, and despair. However, it's crucial to recognize the powerful influence of negativity bias, the tendency to dwell on negative information. This bias can cause us to fixate on worst-case scenarios, blinding us to the glimmers of hope that persist.

Extensive research has shown that negative thinking has far-reaching consequences for our health, weakening our immune system, elevating the risk of serious conditions like hypertension, heart disease, and stroke, and contributing to a host of other health problems, from diabetes and obesity to depression, anxiety, migraines, and chronic pain. Moreover, contemplating or visualizing adverse outcomes triggers harmful stress responses, releasing cortisol and adrenaline, which further exacerbate health issues and take a toll on our mental and emotional well-being, fostering anxiety, hopelessness, and despair.

When facing a chronic illness, it's easy to become fixated on physical limitations, the potential impact on our relationships and careers, and the burden of treatments and mortality. These negative thoughts can amplify feelings of hopelessness, depression, and anxiety, possibly even worsening the course of the illness. While acknowledging the challenges is important, it's equally vital to focus on resilience, positivity, and the potential for a better future, for these forces can propel us toward healing and well-being.

Visualization is a powerful tool that can help us overcome negativity bias and create a more supportive environment for healing. When we visualize ourselves as healed and healthy, we generate positive emotions such as hope, joy, and gratitude. These emotions create a fertile ground for healing and transformation within our bodies.

In addition, visualization can help us take an active role in our healing journey. By focusing on the positive, we can shift from the limitations imposed by our health challenges to the boundless possibilities of a healed existence. This shift in perspective can empower us to make the necessary changes to our lives and create the reality we desire.

To practice visualization:

- Find a quiet place where you will not be disturbed.

- Close your eyes and take a few deep breaths to relax.

- Once relaxed, visualize yourself in a desired state and create a clear mental image. When you envision something, you engage the same brain regions that are activated when you actually experience that event. As you visualize, pay attention to all of the details. What do you see? What do you hear? What do you smell? What do you feel?

The more vivid your visualization is, the more effective it will be. Research indicates that the brain treats visualization as a real experience, and it can profoundly impact various cognitive, emotional, and physiological processes. The more vivid and immersive the visualization, the more powerful its effects can be.

Visualization played a pivotal role in my healing journey. By consistently engaging in positive visualizations of myself healed, I was able to stay positive and generate a cascade of uplifting emotions, such as hope, joy, and gratitude. These emotions created a fertile ground for healing and transformation within my body.

Visualization empowered me to take an active role in my healing. It allowed me to shift my focus from the limitations imposed by my health challenges to the boundless possibilities of a healed existence.

If you struggle to overcome negativity bias, try visualization. It is a powerful way to help you shift your focus to the positive and create a more fulfilling life. This simple yet effective tool can help you take an active role in your healing journey and create the reality you desire. Visualize for at least 5–10 minutes daily, each day adding more detail. The more you practice visualization, the more powerful it will become. Journal your discoveries.

Additional Tips for Overcoming Negativity Bias

- Be mindful of your thoughts. Pay attention to the negative thoughts that pop into your head and challenge them. Ask yourself if there is any evidence to support these thoughts.

- Focus on the positive. When you catch yourself having a negative thought, create a positive one to replace it. For example, instead of thinking, "I'm going to be exhausted all day today," state, "I've rested well, and I'm going to feel great today!"

- Surround yourself with positive people. The people you spend time with can significantly impact your outlook on life. Make an effort to spend time with people who are optimistic and supportive.

- Practice gratitude. Taking the time to appreciate the good things in your life, big and small, can help counteract the effects of negativity bias. Try keeping a gratitude journal or taking a few minutes each day to think about what you're grateful for.

Healing Through Divination Tools

Each morning, I seek inner insight with my cherished reflective card deck. With each shuffle and draw, I welcome broader understanding and inspiration into my life.

Some days I ask, "How may I serve today?" and other days I'll ask, "What do I need to know today?" or another question that supports my healing path. Beyond a mere card, this profound tool becomes a doorway to introspection and self-discovery, guiding me to explore the depths of my thoughts and emotions. With pen in hand and a sense of guiding inspiration, I embark on a self-reflective journaling journey that fosters gratitude, mindfulness, and personal growth.

Divination tools are objects or systems used to gain insight. While they are commonly associated with predicting future events, divination tools can also be used as a supportive means for healing and personal growth.

Here's how they can support the healing process:

- *Self-reflection:* Divination tools, such as oracle cards, runes, or pendulums, can act as mirrors that reflect your inner thoughts, emotions, and subconscious patterns. They visually represent your current state, allowing you to explore and reflect on various aspects of your life. This self-reflection can help you better understand yourself, your emotions, and your experiences, leading to personal growth and healing.

- *Increased awareness:* Divination tools can help you become more attuned to your intuition and inner wisdom. Engaging with a divination tool teaches you to trust your instincts and develop a stronger connection with your inner self. This heightened awareness can bring clarity to unresolved issues, allowing you to address them and work toward healing and growth.

- *Empowerment and decision-making:* Divination tools can empower us by offering guidance and insights into different situations. They can help you explore various options and potential outcomes, giving you a fresh perspective on your challenges. This newfound clarity can assist you in making decisions that align with your values and support your healing journey.

- *Emotional support:* Using divination tools can provide emotional support during difficult times. The process of seeking guidance and receiving insights can be comforting and reassuring. Divination tools can offer solace, encouragement, and validation.

- *Symbolic language:* Divination tools often employ symbols, archetypes, and metaphors to convey meaning. These symbolic representations can tap into your subconscious mind, bypassing rational thinking and connecting with deeper layers of understanding. They can help you uncover hidden patterns, unresolved emotions, and underlying causes of imbalance or discomfort, supporting healing and transformation.

- *Ritual and mindfulness:* Divination tools can be a ritual or mindfulness practice. A regular divination practice is sacred self-care. It encourages you to slow down, be present in the moment, and cultivate a deeper connection with yourself. This intentional practice can promote relaxation, reduce stress, and contribute to healing.

Divination tools should be approached with an open and discerning mindset. While they can offer valuable insights and support, they are not definitive answers or a substitute for professional help. They can complement other healing modalities, such as therapy or counseling, by providing an additional perspective and promoting self-awareness.

SoulCollage®: An Artful Path to Self-Discovery and Healing

SoulCollage® is a creative and intuitive process that involves creating personal collaged cards for self-expression, self-discovery, and healing. (For disclosure's sake, let me mention that I'm a professional SoulCollage facilitator myself.) Here's how SoulCollage cards can support the healing process:

- *Self-exploration:* Creating SoulCollage cards provides a creative outlet for self-expression. By selecting images, arranging them, and collaging them onto cards, you tap into your subconscious mind and explore your thoughts, feelings, desires, and experiences. Through this process, you gain insights into your inner world, uncovering hidden aspects of yourself and promoting self-awareness.

- *Integration and wholeness:* SoulCollage cards often represent different aspects of your personality, emotions, memories, and dreams. By creating and working with these cards, you can integrate and honor all these parts of yourself. It allows you to embrace your complexities, contradictions, and strengths, fostering a sense of wholeness and self-acceptance. This integration can be a powerful catalyst for healing and personal growth.

- *Healing trauma and emotional wounds:* SoulCollage cards can be beneficial for healing trauma and emotional wounds. As you create and engage with the cards, you may uncover symbols, images, or themes that resonate with your past experiences. Utilizing SoulCollage cards in a secure and nurturing setting, with a therapist's or social worker's guidance, can play a significant role in promoting healing. It offers a valuable avenue for examining, processing, and releasing challenging emotions and traumatic memories.

- *Externalizing inner dialogues:* SoulCollage cards can be a tool for externalizing and exploring inner dialogues. You can create cards representing different aspects of yourself, relationships, or situations and engage in a conversation between the cards. This process allows a deeper understanding of conflicting emotions, inner conflicts, and unresolved issues. By giving these aspects a voice, you can gain clarity, resolve conflicts, and work toward healing and resolution.

- *Reflection and insight:* SoulCollage cards serve as visual reminders of your inner journey and growth. By regularly reflecting on and journaling about your cards, you deepen your understanding of their symbolism and messages. The process of contemplation and interpretation can bring about valuable insights, providing guidance, inspiration, and a deeper connection to your inner wisdom.

- *Community and support:* SoulCollage can be practiced individually or in groups. Joining a SoulCollage community or workshop provides a supportive environment for sharing and witnessing each other's cards and stories. The collective experience and feedback can offer validation, encouragement, and a sense of belonging—essential elements of the healing process.

I became a SoulCollage facilitator because I wanted to share the profound healing that this process imparts. Witnessing the transformative effects of SoulCollage in my own life, I was inspired to guide others on their paths of healing and self-exploration. Being a SoulCollage facilitator is immensely rewarding; I have witnessed firsthand its profound impact on individuals' lives, helping them heal, grow, and connect with their authentic selves.

SoulCollage is a personal and intuitive process; there are no "right" or "wrong" ways to create or interpret the cards. It is a unique and individual journey that allows you to access your inner wisdom and navigate your healing path.

Visit the official SoulCollage website at www.soulcollage.com to locate facilitators in your area.

Self-Help Books for Introspection and Healing

- *The Road Less Traveled: A New Psychology of Love, Traditional Values, and Spiritual Growth*, Dr. M. Scott Peck

- *Love: What Life Is All About*, Leo Buscaglia

- *You Can Heal Your Life*, Louise L. Hay

- *The Key to Self-Liberation*, Christiane Beerlandt

- *Change Your Thoughts, Change Your Life: Living the Wisdom of the Tao*, Dr. Wayne W. Dyer

- *The Magic*, Rhonda Byrne

- *The Journey: A Practical Guide to Healing Your Life and Setting Yourself Free*, Brandon Bays

- *SoulCollage Evolving: An Intuitive Collage Process for Self-Discovery and Community*, Seena B. Frost

- *Loving What Is: Four Questions That Can Change Your Life*, Byron Katie

Chapter 12

RESEARCH Q & A

Motivated by my experience with lupus decades ago and a keen interest in understanding progress since then, I've compiled the following series of questions and answers informed by current research.

 ## What is lupus?

Lupus is a chronic inflammatory autoimmune disease with a wide range of clinical presentations resulting from its effect on multiple organ systems. There are four main types of lupus: neonatal, discoid, drug-induced, and systemic lupus erythematosus (SLE), the type that affects the majority of patients. Patients with lupus experience a loss of self-tolerance as a result of abnormal immunological function and the production of autoantibodies, which lead to the formation of immune complexes that may adversely affect healthy tissue.[1]

Although the precise etiologic mechanism is unknown, genetic, hormonal, and environmental factors, as well as immune abnormalities, have been identified. Associations between lupus onset and age, sex, geography, and race have also been established. Management of this disease should be individualized and should include both pharmacological and nonpharmacological modalities for symptom relief and resolution as well as improved quality of life.[1]

Lupus is associated with multisystemic inflammation resulting from abnormal immunological function. Patients experience periodic flares of varying severity or instances in which no observable signs or symptoms are present.

What are the main classifications of lupus?

There are four main types of lupus:[1,5]

- *Systemic Lupus Erythematosus (SLE)* is an autoimmune disease in immunological function. It is characterized by autoantibodies, immune complex formation, and immune dysregulation, resulting in damage.[5]

- *Discoid Lupus Erythematosus (DLE)* is a "chronic, scarring, atrophy producing, photosensitive dermatosis. The pathophysiology of DLE may be suggested as a heat shock protein induced in the keratinocyte following UV light exposure or stress, and this protein may act as a target for T-cell mediated epidermal cell cytotoxicity."[5]

- *Drug-induced Lupus* is a lupus-like autoimmune disorder, which usually happens after months or years of prolonged exposure to specific medicines, and that goes away after the offending prescription is stopped.[12]

- *Neonatal Lupus Erythematosus (NLE)* is a syndrome of clinical symptoms found in newborns of mothers who have antibodies to soluble nuclear antigens.[13]

How does lupus develop?

As the understanding of the development of SLE is constantly evolving, its pathogenesis or development is complex. When genetically susceptible individuals get exposed to environmental factors, the break in tolerance leads to autoimmunity.[4] The immune system cannot determine "self," so it attacks one's cells, leading to SLE.[2]

Technically, cell damage makes the immune system vulnerable to self-antigens, causing T- and B-cell activation, which triggers a sustained, self-aimed immune response. Cytokine release, complement activation, and autoantibody production damages the organs.[4]

What are the factors associated with lupus onset?

Since there is no specific cause of SLE identified,[5] some factors (i.e., genes, environment, and hormones) have been defined to affect numerous elements of both innate and adaptive immune responses.[6] These factors are highly associated with the onset of SLE, especially to those with a predisposition by heredity[3] or race[7] of lupus. As discussed in the following paragraphs, it appears that there is a heritable component to lupus. It is more likely that lupus will occur to those who are descendants of lupus patients. This is why doctors examine the clinical history of not only the person being diagnosed but also their ancestry. It's possible that the genetic factor related to lupus will remain dormant unless environmental factors (sun, smoking, drugs, etc.) trigger them.

Race

Non-Caucasians are more susceptible to lupus. The majority of lupus patients are from African, Latin, or Asian ancestry.[6]

Genes

A heritable component has been long-recognized in SLE.[1] Comprehensive studies and meta-analyses of genome-wide association have determined close to 150 new SLE risk loci across different ancestries, proving that genetic and epigenetic factors directly correlate to alteration of innate and adaptive immune systems.[6] It is recognized that there is a higher risk of developing SLE (and other immune disease) among relatives.[3] The genetically determined heritability was calculated at 43.90%.[3]

Environment

Ultraviolet radiation, smoking, and drugs are well-established environmental factors linked to the onset of lupus. At least 118 drugs have been associated with induced lupus, particularly procainamide and hydralazine, while anti-tumor necrosis factor agents (infliximab, adalimumab, etanercept) have been linked to anti-DNA antibody production.[3] Other environmental triggers include viruses such as the Epstein-Barr virus, low vitamin D levels, and environmental pollutants.[1] Recently, COVID-19 has been found to trigger the onset of SLE.[8]

Hormones

Besides influencing the reproductive system, sex hormones regulate the development and function of the immune response.[9] Estrogen affects the lower limit for B-cell apoptosis and activation. While fresh evidence suggests different molecular mechanisms and the likely activation of X-chromosome-defined genes that are genetically connected to SLE, we still don't know why women make up the great majority of persons with SLE or the exact molecular mechanism by which women regulate the immune system.[6]

What life events are associated with the onset of lupus?

Childhood physical and emotional abuse.

A 2021 paper observed that there is a significant increase in risk of SLE among women who suffered physical and emotional abuse in their childhood. Thus, exposure to childhood afflictions may contribute to SLE development.[10]

Stressful life events.

The death of a loved one, guilt, sexual abuse, and divorce that relates to depression are stressful life situations known to contribute to SLE development.[11]

How is lupus diagnosed?

The diagnosis of SLE is composed of typical clinical manifestations and positive serologies. Lupus patients present a heterogenous clinical manifestations leading to the creation of numerous sets of classification criteria over time for epidemiological and research purposes.[14]

How does one receive a confirmed lupus diagnosis?

SLE is diagnosed clinically, with test abnormalities such as serologic assays supporting the diagnosis. SLE has no diagnostic criteria, hence classification criteria are frequently employed instead, but with significant drawbacks. The EULAR/ACR-2019 classification criteria provides the best combination of sensitivity and specificity among classification criteria, although they require a positive antinuclear antibody (ANA) as an admission condition.[3]

These classification criteria take into account different symptoms of lupus. The American Rheumatism Association Committee on Diagnostic and Therapeutic Criteria recognizes oral or nasopharyngeal ulcers as a key diagnostic symptom of SLE.[5]

Diagnosis can be difficult in three situations: (1) early stages of the disease, when only a few symptoms are evident; (2) ANA-negative instances or organ-dominant types; and (3) rare disease presentations, which can be severe and require immediate treatment.[3]

A study by Sloan[15] showed that the average time from first experiencing symptoms of lupus/connective tissue diseases (CTD) to diagnosis was 6 years, 11 months (mean) and 4 years (median). Notably, 24% of patients reported that a diagnosis took more than 10 years while 22% reported a diagnosis within a year.

Some factors may delay the diagnosis. Non-specific general changes (fatigue, weight loss, subfebrile states) as well as clinical symptoms that have developed within months, or even years, may hamper a diagnosis.[16]

 ## Is a lupus test available?

Lupus has many manifestations and symptoms vary from one patient to another. Thus, no single test can diagnose lupus, so a classification criterion was developed. The diagnosis of SLE is clinical, supported by laboratory investigation indicative of immune reactivity or inflammation in various organs. Along with symptoms and signs, the sets of classification criteria use blood tests, urine tests, and skin or renal biopsies to confirm diagnosis.[3] Thus, the question of which is the most accurate is misleading, because clinical manifestations of lupus are heterogenous (not a uniform set of symptoms/manifestations among all cases), and doctors need every test applicable before accurately diagnosing lupus.

Blood tests

The blood tests used in lupus diagnosis include an ANA test, anti-DNA antibody test, anti-Sm antibody test, serum (blood) complement test, and complement proteins C3 and C4 test.[5] A positive ANA is seen in more than 97% of cases of SLE. However, it can also be seen in several other disorders and a significant proportion of the healthy population, and has a specificity of only 20%. Hence, a positive ANA does not confirm SLE diagnosis, but a negative ANA makes it significantly less likely. Complements C3 and C4 are typically checked in patients with SLE or suspicion of SLE, and low complement levels indicate complement consumption and may correlate with disease activity. Markers of inflammation such as erythrocyte sedimentation rate and C-reactive protein may be elevated.[4]

Urine tests and biopsies

Renal involvement is a common and major symptom of SLE, affecting up to 60% of adult SLE patients and up to 80% of pediatric SLE patients.[17] Thus, urine tests or a biopsy may be done.

Renal biopsy is still the gold standard for measuring lupus nephritis activity and is useful in determining therapy response.[17-18] Renal biopsy is performed if there is a suspicion of lupus nephritis.

Skin biopsies can be considered, especially if there is an atypical presentation.[4] Given the invasive nature of biopsies, which pose a significant risk of complications, particularly in children, there is a continuing search for non-invasive methods.[17] A biopsy can also be done to the skin for the diagnosis of cutaneous lupus or skin involvement.[14]

Urine is a great biomarker source, since it can be collected non-invasively and contains fewer proteins than blood.[17] A laboratory-based urine test was successfully established for early diagnosis of SLE patients, with sensitivity and specificity measurements of these biomarkers ranging from 53-100% and 50-71%, respectively, among all SLE patients. 72% of the possible urine biomarkers for SLE could be detected using tandem mass spectrometry.[19]

Other tests

Other lab tests involved include chest imaging with computed tomography (CT) scan, cardiac workup including echocardiography (trans-esophageal when suspecting Libman-Sacks endocarditis), CNS workup with magnetic resonance imaging (MRI), and/or lumbar puncture if specific organ involvement is suspected.[4]

 ## How do patients react to lupus when diagnosed?

A lupus diagnosis stimulates different reactions from patients. Surprisingly, relief is a common reaction of patients to the diagnosis.[16] Patients become frustrated and anxious due to long diagnosis processes, illness courses with few or modest symptoms, non-specific symptoms (weakness, fatigue), and questions from loved ones and even doctors about the veracity of reported symptoms. They become calmer after receiving a diagnosis and a chance to begin treatment.[16]

Others experience stress and anxiety in response to the diagnosis. Unpredictable disease progression can instill worry and a sense of uneasiness about one's future. Some patients' responses are denial. They appear to not understand the diagnosis because they undervalue it.[16]

How does lupus affect each organ system?

Lupus displays different organ manifestations. New developments have come into the light over time. The following are the effects of lupus on each organ system.[14]

Skin

Photosensitive distribution is a major feature of cutaneous lupus. It is important to distinguish cutaneous lupus from other, more prevalent photosensitive rashes such as polymorphous light eruption or rosacea. A non-lupus cause, such as non-specific inflammatory reactions or polymorphous light eruption, is ultimately found in more than 50% of "photosensitive" biopsied rashes in SLE patients. In lupus, a real photosensitive rash is elevated, delayed, and persistent.[14]

The sun is very much still a concern. Sun exposure causes an increase in cell apoptosis, which is known to cause SLE as well as its exacerbation and flares. It often starts days after exposure to ultraviolet light, lasts for longer than three weeks, and may be accompanied by systemic symptoms such arthralgia or fatigue.[14]

Hair

SLE frequently includes alopecia, which can have a variety of causes. True lupus alopecia, often known as "lupus hair," is reversible and is defined by the frontal hair becoming shorter, more erratic, and filled with broken hairs between five and twenty-five millimeters in length. Lupus with lifelong scarring can develop from discoid lupus. Smoking raises the likelihood of discoid lupus, increases continuing cutaneous activity, and reduces the effectiveness of hydroxychloroquine, all of which are risk factors for SLE.[14]

Joint/musculoskeletal involvement

At some point over the course of their illness, 80 to 90 percent of SLE patients experience musculoskeletal symptoms, which can vary from minor arthralgias to deforming arthritis. Although any joint can be affected, lupus arthritis mainly affects tiny joints in the hands, knees, and wrists. It is a non-erosive, symmetrical inflammatory polyarthritis. The non-erosive abnormalities of the hands, such as ulnar deviation and subluxation of the metacarpophalangeal joints, which may resemble rheumatoid arthritis, are caused by the joint capsule and ligament laxity in Jaccoud's arthropathy. These abnormalities are often reducible, yet they sporadically might become fixed.[4]

Kidneys

About 50% of lupus patients have renal involvement, with some racial groups, such as African-Americans, being more susceptible (70%).[14] The most frequent reason for kidney damage in people with systemic lupus erythematosus, and a significant risk factor for morbidity and mortality, is lupus nephritis (LN).[20] Within ten years of diagnosis, up to 60% of SLE patients develop lupus nephritis.[1]

Since lupus nephritis is a leading cause of morbidity and death in SLE and delayed identification increases the likelihood of end-stage renal disease, early detection and treatment are essential. When there is proteinuria, renal disease is thought to be present. However, 25% of SLE patients may have lupus nephritis (class III, IV, or V) without any obvious indications of renal illness. A renal biopsy should be performed if the urine protein level is above 500 mg per 24 hours, which is linked to histopathological lupus nephritis.[14]

Central nervous system

SLE has been linked to a wide range of neuropsychiatric symptoms. Nevertheless, only a small number of them are more specific for SLE and useful for diagnosis. They include seizures, psychosis, multiple mononeuritis, myelitis, peripheral or cranial neuropathy, and acute confusional condition (delirium). Importantly, this demands ruling out other established reasons. Intractable headaches, which are recorded in more than 50% of the cases examined by Justiz, are the most typical CNS manifestation.[14]

Cardiovascular manifestations

Any layer of the heart, such as the pericardium, myocardium, endocardium, and even the coronary arteries, may be affected by SLE. The most frequent cardiac symptom is pericarditis with exudative pericardial effusions. Antiphospholipid antibody syndrome may be related to valvular anomalies, particularly Libman-Sacks endocarditis affecting the mitral valve. Due to coronary vasculitis or, more frequently, widespread atherosclerosis, patients with SLE are more at risk for developing coronary artery disease.[4]

What are the current trends in lupus?

Prevalence

Between 20 to 150 instances per 100,000 individuals are reported, and this prevalence looks to be rising as more people become aware of the illness and survival rates rise.[6]

Races

People with African, Hispanic, or Asian heritage in the United States are likely to have higher rates of SLE and more severe organ involvement than people of other races or ethnicities.[6]

Mortality

The annual age-standardized mortality rate is currently 2.7 deaths per million inhabitants. Women experience 4.5 fatalities per million people while men experience 0.8 deaths per million people.[20] The ten-year survival rate has dramatically increased over the last 50 years to more than 70%, mostly due to increased knowledge of the illness, the widespread and prudent use of immunosuppressive medications, and a more effective approach to treating infections, the primary cause of death.[6] Infection and cardiovascular disease are the two leading causes of death worldwide, and both of these conditions can likely be reduced with higher-quality medical care.[20]

Investigations of the causes of death in SLE patients have also been conducted using the National Center for Health Statistics' multiple cause of death database. According to this data, the most common conditions among deceased female SLE patients were sepsis (4.3%) and hypertension (3.0%), whereas the most common conditions among deceased male SLE patients were cardiac disease (3.7%) and complications from diabetes mellitus (3.6%).[21]

The death rate associated with SLE is still high despite breakthroughs in treatment. It is particularly alarming that mortality in developed nations has not decreased recently. The overall chance of survival is 95% five years after diagnosis, 91% after ten years, 85% after fifteen years, and 78% after twenty years. Early death is frequently linked to infection and active disease, whereas late mortality is frequently attributed to damage, corticosteroid-mediated harm, and cardiovascular disease.[1]

Average lifespan

SLE patients continue to experience unacceptably high rates of mortality, two to three times greater than those of the general population.[20] Women with SLE die on average 22 years earlier than women without SLE among deceased patients (median age of death for SLE patients is 59 years against 81 years for those without SLE), but this difference is just 12 years for male patients (median age of death for patients with SLE 61 years versus 73 years for those without SLE).[21]

Percentage of abled to work vs. long-term disability

According to a recent study,[22] 25% of SLE patients become specifically work-handicapped at five years and 50% at ten years due to the disease. Additionally, job disability is more closely related to socioeconomic position and a lower self-reported quality of life than it is to disease symptoms and co-morbidities. The cumulative rate of job disability (standard error) is 5% (0.018) at one year, 25% (0.039) at five years, and 54% (0.058) at ten years. The National Institute of Statistics and Census conducted the most recent study in Argentina in 2018, and it found that 11.8 percent of the population who were employed had any kind of persistent handicap, with 55.4 percent of them being unemployed.[22]

Number of people with lupus in the world today

There are five million people with SLE in the world today.[23] Global estimates of the prevalence and incidence of SLE in adults range from 30 to 150 per 100,000 and 2.2 to 23.1 per 100,000, respectively.[1] This is an increased number compared to the last 40 years since milder cases are being more recognized.[3]

Women vs. men

Nearly ten women suffer with SLE for every man who contracts the illness, a notable female predominance.[3] The female-to-male ratio in women between the ages of 15 and 44 reaches up to 13:1, whereas it is just 2:1 in young children and the elderly.[14] While rare, lupus symptoms tend to be worse in men compared to women.[4]

Country of highest cases

The US has the highest number of lupus cases, mostly because it's the most documented country in terms of lupus. Studies strongly point out that North America has the most incidents of lupus (between 3.7 and 49 per 100,000 persons) while Africa has the most prevalence (between 601.3 and 7,713.5 per 100,000 persons).[21] The widely used estimate is 1.5 million cases in the US. However, using the sex- and race-specific prevalence estimates to the proportionate stratum-specific population denominators from 2018 U.S. Census data, and only an estimated number of 204,295 persons in the US fulfilled American College of Rheumatology criteria for SLE.[24]

Age of onset

Age is one of the most important factors influencing lupus patients' clinical symptoms and prognosis. Lupus can develop at any age, but it is most common during the reproductive years. The average age of diagnosis in adults is 24 to 32 years, while in pediatric cases it is 12 to 17 years.[25]

 ## What are the most common complaints of lupus sufferers?

Fatigue, joint pain, and photosensitivity.[26]

 ## What is the cost per patient per year to stay on lupus medications in the US?

Annual direct (health-care-related) costs in the United States for lupus are estimated to be between $3,000 and $12,000 (2018 estimates), depending on the severity of the disease and organ(s) involved.[3] As of 2021, according to the Lupus Foundation of America, the annual costs before the diagnosis are $12,373 for people with mild lupus,

$22,559 for people with moderate lupus, and $39,261 for people with severe lupus. Following the diagnosis, the annual healthcare costs rise to $13,415 for those with mild lupus, $29,512 for those with moderate lupus, and $68,260 for those with severe lupus.[27]

What is a day in the life of a lupus patient like?

A study[28] by de Souza et al., entitled *Duality of Living with SLE: Fluctuating Between "Good Days" and "Bad Days,"* explored the lives of 26 lupus patients. Patients have a common set of manifestations: tiredness, fatigue, arthritis, pain, edema in the upper and lower limbs, Sjogren's syndrome, and other skin manifestations. It turns out that living with lupus isn't a crystallized experience. It is composed of good and bad days. Good days relate to periods of low disease activity or remission. Bad days relate to exacerbations or flares.

For a lupus patient, every tomorrow is a mystery. On a good day, patients feel fine and are able to carry out tasks just like everyone else. On a bad day, however, they feel worse and are unable to carry out tasks. It's hard to walk, do chores, go to work, or much else. They get tired often and feelings of stress, frustration and fear all come into the picture. If they exert themselves one day, they suffer in pain and fatigue for many days to follow. Living with lupus is living in isolation. The feeling of constant tiredness prohibits patients to go out. They spend their time idly during the worst days.[28]

Medications are a big part of a patient's daily routine. Patients also have to schedule appointments with their doctors. These come with worry due to the financial burden they cause. This feeling of being a burden adds up to the negative emotional impact of lupus.[16]

At night, nearly 95% of patients suffer from sleep disorders. This comes as a result of pain, stress, depression, treatment side effects, and physical changes caused by lupus. Thus, sleep hardly eases fatigue.[16]

At some point during the course of the disease, patients will accept the disease and find a way of coping. Staying optimistic and maintaining an active life is usually the mechanism patients find effective.[16] Nonetheless, professional, social, and family support is as important to positively affect daily life.[28]

What are patients' limitations and how has having lupus changed their lives?

Lupus influences many facets of patients' lives, including how they deal with stress, their intimate relationships, their work and home-related activities, and their treatment adherence. They frequently face varying degrees of physical and mental limitations; they can deal with these limitations by either intentionally minimizing their impact (coping) or maximizing it (catastrophizing).[29]

Fatigue basically forces patients to resign early from hobbies, chores, work, or other family or personal responsibilities like parenthood or medication adherence. They can work up to a certain point, but their productivity and physical activity in general is greatly decreased. Photosensitivity prohibits patients to leave the house. Other factors such as skin manifestations and appearance issues affect their self-image and effectively put them on isolation from everybody else.[29]

A higher catastrophizing score associates a poor mental health, which can imply two things. Catastrophizing is increased by lower health-related quality of life (HRQoL), which intensifies pain and depression and further lowers the patient's HRQoL. In terms of intimate relationships, while a stronger HRQoL is linked to a better sexual function, women with SLE have lower sexual function than healthy controls.[29]

The association between HRQoL and work disability is bidirectional; greater HRQoL enables the patient to work, which in turn improves the patient's mood. Poorer HRQoL, particularly its physical component, is related with work disability. Poor HRQoL is also linked to decreased activity, work productivity, and ADLs; frequently, patients may require assistance from friends and/or family.[29]

 ## What is the effect of lupus on families?

Family and social relationships are negatively impacted by lupus. Due to ongoing fatigue and bad moods, lupus patients neglect their household and family tasks. Women frequently express worry that they lack the strength to care for children, disregard their responsibilities as wives and hosts, and neglect their motherly, domestic, and marital responsibilities. When relatives try to absolve them of their responsibilities, the patient may become irritated and frustrated because they feel helpless and powerless.[16]

Some individuals choose to continue working despite the disease's symptoms because they wish to keep their independence. Patients cite carrying heavy objects, doing laundry, shopping, and looking after children as the most difficult tasks. Patients are able to avoid carrying an excessive burden thanks to the family's appropriate support.[16]

Patients who are married or have a life partner have been found to have higher HRQoL than single people. It is unclear, though, whether this is because partners provide greater support or because people with low HRQoL are less likely to form relationships. Patients worry that they may burden the family because of their growing infirmity. They become uninterested in regular life activities due to fatigue and melancholy.[16]

As patients spend less time with their partners (who consequently have more duties), the condition has a negative effect on relationships as well. Patients fear being rejected and cut off. Young patients worry that they won't meet a partner who will accept their illness and that they won't be able to have children. Patients' social lives are restricted because of the unpredictable course of SLE.[16]

Because some symptoms, including weariness, are "invisible," friends may not understand why patients cancel appointments. Patients who are photosensitive frequently have to say no to spending time with their relatives (activities in the open air, going to the beach). They become more isolated as a result, which irritates them.[16]

What is the positive effect of lupus on patients?

It's hard to adjust and accept lupus, especially for younger people who have so much life ahead of them. It takes time. With the difficulties, uncertainties and domineering aspects of the disease come new priorities. Amazingly, patients find positivity in light of the inconveniences and limitations of the disease. They develop awareness of their bodies and disease. They become more resilient and learn how to live with the disease and "overcome the obstacles of everyday life." They learn to be more grateful and joyful to the simple pleasures of life. Lupus also makes them realize the things they want to do and resign from those they don't. It becomes an avenue to make valuable connections, old and new. They begin to focus on what matters.[16]

What effect does pregnancy have on lupus?

Most women with lupus can have successful pregnancies, and there are steps that may be taken to lower the risks of poor outcomes for either the mother or the fetus.[3] Positive antiphospholipid antibodies in SLE patients increase the risk of pre-eclampsia, maternal thrombosis, spontaneous abortions, and fetal loss. Neonatal lupus, which manifests as a photosensitive rash, cytopenia, and transaminitis, can result from anti-Ro (SSA) and anti-La (SSB) antibodies crossing the placenta. If there is a history of neonatal lupus in a previous pregnancy, the risk rises to 20% from 2% during the first pregnancy.[4]

SLE frequently flares during pregnancy, particularly if the condition was uncontrolled in the six months prior to conception. Although various clinical and laboratory characteristics (low complements, positive Anti-Ds-DNA antibody, normal serum uric acid level, and active urine sediment) may aid, it can be difficult to distinguish lupus nephritis from pre-eclampsia. Particularly at a very high risk of mortality during pregnancy are those with more severe SLE signs, such as pulmonary hypertension, serious cardiovascular illness, or cerebrovascular accident.[4]

 ## Is it advised that a lupus patient not get pregnant?

Some SLE patients completely give up growing their families and becoming parents out of worry that their children may develop the illness as well. Since lupus aggravation affects nearly half of patients during pregnancy, some women choose to have an abortion. In the course of SLE, pregnancy problems and fetal malformations occur more frequently than in the general population. Preparing the patient for pregnancy and ensuring ongoing monitoring throughout the process are therefore crucial.[16]

 ## What effect do vaccines have on lupus patients?

No licensed vaccines that are currently recommended have been proven to play a part in the development of SLE.[30] Live vaccines should generally be avoided in patients receiving significant immunosuppression, but important exceptions to this rule are the measles, mumps, and rubella (MMR) and varicella vaccines.[30]

Are lupus patients advised against taking COVID-19 vaccines?

Indeed, there may be a higher risk of hospitalization and death for SLE patients with COVID-19 compared to the general population, probably with a greater risk for those patients who are taking rituximab, according to studies looking at outcomes to date. The immunization against COVID-19 will be crucial for those with SLE, even if it is vital to interpret these data with caution.

Since none of the COVID-19 vaccines now approved for use in emergencies are live-attenuated vaccines, the historical practice of avoiding live-attenuated immunizations for many SLE patients is no longer relevant. The vaccines from AstraZeneca/Oxford and Janssen, which use non-replicating viral vectors, are regarded as safe for those with immunodeficiencies.[30]

Are any lupus cures documented?

There is no cure for lupus.[4,31] While no cure has ever been found, researchers are continually looking for treatments. Lupus is considered a chronic disease without cure. Certainly, researchers are focused on different medications that can minimize the disease activity.[1]

What are the current treatments for lupus?

Since no cure has been found yet, the goals of lupus treatment are:[14]

- Maintain lowest degree of activity using immunomodulators, immunosuppression as appropriate and avoiding known triggers.

- Prevent organ damage from active lupus.

- Reduce comorbidities secondary to lupus and its treatment, especially accelerated atherosclerosis, the major cause of death.

- Address the fatigue and pain associated with lupus.

It is crucial to begin treatment as soon as possible and work together with the patient to achieve these common objectives. This entails avoiding known flare-up-inducing factors, the requirement for sun protection, the maximization of immunomodulators (hydroxychloroquine and vitamin D, including adherence monitoring), avoiding the use of maintenance prednisone >6 mg daily, and, as necessary, controlling active disease with immunosuppression or biologics.[14] As discussed in the following, some therapies have negative side effects.

Immunomodulators

Without raising the danger of infection or cancer, immunomodulators can effectively control the immune system in SLE patients.

Hydroxychloroquine

Prescription: Hydroxychloroquine PO 200–400 mg daily.[5] Adverse effects: The danger of infection or cancer is not increased by hydroxychloroquine and it's non-immunosuppressive.[14] However, it can cause macular damage and muscle weakness.[5]

Vitamin D[14]

Supplementation: Should be aimed to a 25(OH) vitamin D level of 40 ng/ml. Adverse effects: N/A. Vitamin D supplementation is safe and should continue continuously. Vitamin D levels should be regularly evaluated to ensure optimal absorption, dose, and adherence.

Dehydroepiandrosterone (DHEA)

Prescription: 200 mg.[46] Use: DHEA supplementation has been associated with regulation of proinflammatory cytokines. In women with lupus, there is a consistent pattern of lower androgen levels, higher estradiol, and reduced levels of both DHEA and its metabolite DHEA-S, irrespective of corticosteroid usage. Adverse effects: Since DHEA may increase the risk of hormone-sensitive cancers, postmenopausal women shouldn't use it. Mild acne or hair growth may result from dehydroepiandrosterone. DHEA use in men is not supported by any evidence.[14]

Corticosteroids

Prescription: For patient quality of life, maintenance dosages of 5 mg or less are unquestionably frequently warranted.[1] Adverse effects/use: As much as possible, oral corticosteroids should be avoided.[14] Many of the infections, damage accumulation, and early mortality in SLE are caused by corticosteroids. When a patient receives an average daily prednisone dose of more than 6 to 12 mg, there is a 50% higher risk of experiencing organ damage.

CYTOTOXIC-IMMUNOSUPPRESSANTS

Cyclophosphamide

Prescription: Since it produces equivalent efficacy but fewer infections than the higher-dose treatment, which is $0.5\text{-}1\text{g/m}^2$ monthly for 6 months for non-responders, 500 mg every 2 weeks for 3 months for the responders.[1] Adverse effects: Premature ovarian failure, hemorrhagic cystitis, a higher chance of bladder and other cancers, leukopenia, and an elevated risk of infections are all connected to cyclophosphamide.[14]

Azathioprine

Prescription: PO 1-3 mg/kg per day.[5] Adverse effects: Hepatotoxicity, malignancy, infertility, myelosuppression, renal failure, and an elevated risk of infection.[14]

Methotrexate

Prescription: 15-20 mg per week. Use: Since it's a teratogen, it can't be used in pregnancy.[14]

Mycophenolate mofetil

Prescription: PO 1-3 g daily. Adverse effects/use: Enteric-coated mycophenolate sodium is an alternative for people who experience gastrointestinal sensitivity to mycophenolate mofetil. Like methotrexate, it is teratogenic, and maternal exposure has been linked to a high rate of fetal losses and a particular pattern of birth abnormalities.[1]

CALCINEURIN INHIBITORS

B-cell drugs[1]

B-cells are involved in T-cell antigen presentation, cytokine release, and the production of autoantibodies; aberrant B-cell pathways are frequently present in SLE.

Belimumab[1]

Belimumab is most helpful when given as a weekly subcutaneous injection or as a monthly intravenous infusion to patients who have high disease activity despite standard therapy, serological abnormalities, and steroid dependence.

Rituximab[1]

Side effect: Reduces vaccine efficacy.[30]

When was the last medication introduced in the US for lupus?

Anifrolumab (anifrolumab-fnia; Saphnelo™) is a monoclonal antibody antagonist of the type 1 interferon receptor (IFNAR). It was developed by AstraZeneca (under license from Medarex, now Bristol-Myers Squibb) for the treatment of autoimmune disorders, including systemic lupus erythematosus (SLE) and lupus nephritis, the underlying pathogenesis of which involves type 1 interferon. In July 2021, intravenous anifrolumab was approved in the US for the treatment of adult patients with moderate to severe SLE who are receiving standard therapy. Anifrolumab (intravenous or subcutaneous) continues to be assessed in clinical studies in SLE in various countries, and the intravenous formulation is under regulatory review in the EU and Japan.[32] There is consistent efficacy and safety of anifrolumab across a range of patients with moderate to severe SLE.[33]

 ## Who are the top lupus researchers?

Expertscape is a reliable website that ranks top experts for medical issues. Based on 21,195 eligible published articles since 2012, the top researchers of lupus worldwide include:[34]

- David Alan Isenberg
- George C. Tsokos
- Michelle A. Petri
- Martin Aringer
- Brad H. Rovin
- Ronald F. van Vollenhoven

- Richard Alan Furie

- Hai-Feng Pan

- Andrea S. Doria

- George K. Bertsias

What have been the outcomes of lupus clinical trials?

Interferon-blocking drugs[1]

The interferon pathway has been studied as a potential therapeutic target in SLE as a result of the discovery of interferonopathies (rare mendelian disorders associated with type 1 interferon overproduction) and the long-standing recognition of an interferon gene signature in many SLE patients, the magnitude of which is correlated with disease activity. Patients without active renal or neurological disease experienced significant improvements in total disease activity, including that of the skin and joints, in a phase 2B trial with the anti-interferon-receptor biological anifrolumab, achieving the LLDAS aim. Patients with strong baseline interferon gene profiles were more affected by this variation than other groups of patients. Phase 3 research is still ongoing.

Other B-cell targets and therapies[1]

The SLE responder index-4 response rate showed a trend toward improvement at week 24, which was most obvious with atacicept 75 mg, even though the study's primary goal was not met. Both the 75 mg and 150 mg groups reduced flare-ups in patients with high disease activity. Patients with high baseline BAFF and APRIL concentrations showed the most decrease in flare in post-hoc analysis. Additionally, the use of several B-cell treatments is becoming more popular. Patients with severe refractory illness were treated with rituximab followed by belimumab in the Synbiose research, a phase 2 proof of concept study. This led to a decrease in neutrophil extracellular traps and serological abnormalities, as well as a remarkable clinical response.

T-cell therapies[1]

T-cell pathways are also abnormal in SLE patients. T-cell treatments have generated interest, although most study results so far have been unsatisfactory. An IL-12 and IL-23 monoclonal antibody is called ustekinumab. Ustekinumab is a drug that may be of relevance in the future since, in a phase 2 research, 60% of participants who received it were categorized as responders, as opposed to 31% of patients who received a placebo (p=00046).

Bruton's tyrosine kinase (BTK) and Janus kinase (JAK) inhibitors[1]

BTK is markedly overexpressed in people with lupus nephritis. The kinase is involved in the activation of monocytes and macrophages as well as intracellular signaling in B-cells. BTK inhibition has demonstrated promise in SLE murine models.

Numerous inflammatory pathways connected to SLE involve JAKs. Baricitinib, a JAK 1 and 2 inhibitor, produced promising outcomes in a phase 2 study, particularly at doses of 4 mg daily. Studies on humans are now being conducted, and tofacitinib, which inhibits JAK 1 and JAK 3, has been studied in murine models.

Proteasome inhibition[1]

Bortezomib, a proteasome inhibitor that targets plasma cells and prevents nuclear factor kappa B activation, is a commonly used medication to treat multiple myeloma. This medication was demonstrated to lessen disease activity, particularly serological abnormalities, with a significant drop in type 1 interferon activity in a small number of individuals with refractory SLE.

Stem-cell therapies[1]

Stem-cell transplantation, whether autologous (from self), haploidentical (partial HLA match and usually from a sibling), or allogeneic (donor, HLA matched, related, or unrelated), offers an opportunity for treatment-free remission. These regimens, in the first instance, involve cyclophosphamide therapy, with various regimens reported. Treatment with cyclophosphamide alone has long been shown to be beneficial in severe life-threatening and organ-threatening SLE. Traynor and colleagues reported myeloablative autologous stem-cell transplantation in seven patients with resolution of serological abnormalities and disease activity. A European study reported 53 cases in whom high-dose cyclophosphamide was followed by autologous peripheral stem-cell transplantation; 66% of patients were in remission at 6 months, although a third of patients subsequently relapsed, with 12 periprocedural deaths. An autologous non-myeloablative hematopoietic stem-cell transplantation regimen was evaluated in 48 patients, using lower doses of cyclophosphamide; 5-year survival was 84%, with a probability of disease-free survival at 5 years of 50%, with two deaths. Mesenchymal (i.e., multipotent stromal cells) stem-cell therapies have been tried, with and without cyclophosphamide, with improvements in disease activity and serological abnormalities. Although promising, these therapies have not been evaluated for SLE in randomized controlled studies, and substantial variations exist in all the reported protocols.

What does remission mean in the medical field?

The definition of remission in the SLE (DORIS) group agreed that overall clinical remission should be defined as having no or minimal disease activity using composite disease activity measures (SLEDAI score of 0, BILAG 2004 score of D and E only, ECLAM score of 0, and a PGA score of 0 or less), whereas complete remission also requires negative serologies (i.e., presence of anti-dsDNA antibodies and low complement).[1]

Composite disease activity measures are utilized for overall disease activity. The same clinical and laboratory tests done to diagnose lupus are used to measure its activity through the classification criteria.[1] SLEDAI is used globally in routine clinical practice. Additionally, it is the primary factor in the SLE Responder Index (SRI4), which is used in clinical studies and to describe states of low disease activity and remission.[34] When SLEDAI scores 0, remission is proved.[3]

 ## How long is a lupus patient typically in remission?

According to the DORIS definition, the Hopkins Cohort's median time in complete and clinical remission is three months. Only 13.2% of people have sustained remission at one year. A state known as lupus low disease activity state (LLDAS) has also been studied; it is indicated by an SLEDAI-2K score of four or less, the absence of major organ activity, the absence of new lupus disease features, a PGA score of one or less, and a prednisone dose of no more than 7.5 mg per day while taking standard maintenance doses of immunosuppressive or biological medications. The median cumulative length of LLDAS in the validation group is one and a half years. Because SLE is a relapsing, remitting disease, remission and LLDAS can happen for varying lengths of time. In the same group, obtaining

LLDAS with 50% of follow-up visits resulted in a 50% reduction in overall organ damage.[1]

 What does a flare specifically mean, and what stimulates it?

A flare is defined in medical literature as a quantifiable increase in disease activity with new or worse clinical signs and symptoms and/or laboratory measurements. SLE flares need to be separated from active but clinically stable disease and from otherwise small fluctuations in disease activity. The assessor must deem this clinically important, usually with at least some consideration of a change or increase in medication. As well as being distinguished from other diseases including infection, medication reaction, and fibromyalgia, which can mimic or coexist with a flare, flares should also be distinguished from increasing organ deterioration.[37]

Flares have been linked to the accumulation of damage and comorbid conditions (including depression and cardiovascular illness), as well as adverse drug reactions, particularly those connected to corticosteroids. From a socioeconomic standpoint, flares are associated with both direct medical costs and a number of indirect costs connected to lost productivity.[36] Lupus may also flare during pregnancy.[4]

 Why are some lupus cases more severe than others?

Race or ancestry
The severity of the disease might vary depending on ancestry and is typically worse in people of African and Latin American descent.[3-4]

Gender
Gender also determines severity of lupus and it shows that although fewer men have lupus, symptoms are worse for them.[4]

Age

Children's SLE tends to be more severe than that of adults, with a higher prevalence of hematologic abnormalities, hepatosplenomegaly, nephritis, and pericarditis. However, it usually develops more slowly and with a more serious serositis, and fewer Raynaud's, malar rash, nephritis, and neuropsychiatric problems in older persons.[4]

Environment

Exposure to the sun, medicines, smoking, and an unhealthy lifestyle can all contribute to the severity of lupus.

Diet

It's widely known that obesity induces inflammation. A high-fat diet plays a role in the pathogenesis of autoimmune diseases. Vitamin D deficiency is often linked to obesity. In general, diet is a very important factor to be considered by patients because it can either make the manifestations of lupus worse or it can help them in the treatment.[37]

Others

SLE, male patients, patients with low complement, positive anti-DNA or aPL antibodies, patients with high interferon (IFN) signature and patients with moderate to high activity indices are more likely to develop severe SLE.[3]

How are lupus foundations and research centers supporting patients?

Lupus foundations and research centers such as the Lupus Foundation of America, the Lupus Research Alliance, and the World Lupus Federation, which are among the most prominent lupus organizations, are all saying the same thing—the end goal of their existence is to end lupus. Finding a lupus cure, however, is still a long way away. Thankfully, these lupus foundations have funded research that sheds light to the many mysteries of lupus. The pathogenesis of lupus, ever-evolving, has become understood more and more over the last 25 years. Many new patient-friendly medications have been introduced recently that are serving patients better. Some new promising research developments that may improve lupus treatment are also coming up over the next few years, such as stem cell therapies.

Lupus foundations and research centers aim to promote lupus awareness over the world. They also sponsor initiatives that help lupus patients to access services online, including consultation, informational resources, and care groups. Many of these foundations have lupus advocates to increase lupus awareness and improve the public understanding of the disease.

According to the latest report of the Lupus Foundation of America, the most prominent among them all, they secured a total of $82 million funding in 2020-2021 from various sources. Almost $25 million of the fund was used for various lupus research such as lupus nephritis. The Lupus Research Alliance spent $15 million in research and $12 million for scientific programs. The amount of money spent on lupus research depends on the size of the foundation, but it is safe to say that lupus research is a multimillion-dollar industry by right.[39-42]

Chapter 13

CLOSING THOUGHTS

Lupus is a persistent journey, a puzzle that's pieced together one day at a time. Each person with lupus faces unique challenges; but together, as a global community, we are relentless in our pursuit of a cure. Remember that even though lupus affects everyone differently, there are universal steps that can aid in this journey of healing and discovery.

First, always trust yourself. Your body is the most sophisticated machine in existence, and it will tell you what it needs. By being true to yourself and embracing your individuality, you are well on your way to charting your own unique healing path.

Choosing self-care and self-compassion is paramount in managing lupus. Acknowledge that you are battling a chronic condition, and allow yourself grace in the journey. Embrace your emotions, express them in healthy ways, and most importantly, forgive yourself and others. This act will remove the shackles that bind you to past hurt and open up pathways to healing.

Show gratitude for each present moment. Despite the pain and challenges, there are always silver linings to be found. Healing is a process that doesn't happen overnight, so be patient with yourself. Invest time and energy in your well-being. Journaling your thoughts and expressing your feelings can be a powerful tool to document your journey and monitor your progress.

Embrace continuous learning and growth. Love and accept yourself unconditionally. Incorporate meditation and mindfulness into your daily routine, nurturing your relationships and seeking support when necessary. Open your heart to new possibilities, and practice patience and persistence on this path.

It's vital to learn to quiet your mind through relaxation techniques and to release negativity, as these can exacerbate your symptoms. Seek professional help if needed, for there is strength in acknowledging when you need a helping hand.

Rest and relaxation are not just luxuries but necessities. Understand your needs and address them proactively. Visualize your future, not just as a patient with lupus, but as a vibrant, healthy, and thriving individual.

Working on healing your wounds, whether physical or emotional, is an integral part of your journey. Explore new experiences and hobbies that bring you joy, and remember that your mindset, belief in yourself, and disciplined action are what you need to heal.

Lastly, zero in on self-reflection and self-discovery. This journey is not just about battling lupus; it's also an opportunity to discover the depths of your strength and resilience.

As we strive toward a world where lupus becomes a thing of the past, remember that each day is a step toward that goal. Lupus does not define you, and your journey is a testament to your strength and resilience.

A cure may be on the horizon, but until then, know that you are not alone, and your lupus family stands with you every step of the way.

ABCs of Healing

Always trust yourself.

Be you!

Choose self-care and self-compassion.

Do what brings you joy.

Embrace your emotions and express them in healthy ways.

Forgive yourself and others.

Gratitude for the present moment.

Heal at your own pace.

Invest in your well-being.

Journal your thoughts and feelings.

Keep learning and growing.

Love and accept yourself unconditionally.

Meditate and practice mindfulness.

Nurture your relationships and seek support.

Open your heart to new possibilities.

Practice patience and persistence.

Quiet your mind through relaxation techniques.

Release negativity and embrace positivity.

Seek professional help if needed.

Take time for rest and relaxation.

Understand and address your needs.

Visualize a healthy and vibrant future.

Work on healing your wounds.

Xplore new experiences and hobbies.

Your mindset, belief in yourself, and disciplined action are what you need to heal.

Zero in on self-reflection and self-discovery.

References

1. Durcan L, O'Dwyer T, Petri M. Management strategies and future directions for systemic lupus erythematosus in adults. The Lancet. 2019 Jun 8;393(10188):2332-43.

2. Moulton VR, Suarez-Fueyo A, Meidan E, Li H, Mizui M, Tsokos GC. Pathogenesis of human systemic lupus erythematosus: a cellular perspective. Trends in molecular medicine. 2017 Jul 1;23(7):615-35.

3. Fanouriakis A, Tziolos N, Bertsias G, Boumpas DT. Update Ⅰn the diagnosis and management of systemic lupus erythematosus. Annals of the rheumatic diseases. 2021 Jan 1;80(1):14-25.

4. Justiz Vaillant AA, Goyal A, Varacallo M. Systemic Lupus Erythematosus. [Updated 2022 Mar 15]. In: StatPearls [Internet]. Treasure Island (FL): StatPearls Publishing; 2022 Jan. Available from: https://www.ncbi.nlm.nih.gov/books/NBK535405/

5. Malathi L, Reshma SA, Anitha N, Masthan KM. Systemic Lupus Erythematosis And Discoid Lupus Erythematosis-An Overview. European Journal of Molecular & Clinical Medicine.;7(5):2020.

6. Tsokos GC. Autoimmunity and organ damage in systemic lupus erythematosus. Nature immunology. 2020 Jun;21(6):605-14.

7. Metry AM, Al Salmi I, Al Balushi F, Yousef MA, Al Ismaili F, Hola A, Hannawi S. Systemic lupus erythematosus: symptoms and signs at initial presentations. Anti-Inflammatory & Anti-Allergy Agents in Medicinal Chemistry (Formerly Current Medicinal Chemistry-Anti-Inflammatory and Anti-Allergy Agents). 2019 Sep 1;18(2):142-50.

8. Zamani B, Moeini Taba SM, Shayestehpour M. Systemic lupus erythematosus manifestation following COVID-19: a case report. Journal of Medical Case Reports. 2021 Dec;15(1):1-4.

9. Moulton VR. Sex hormones in acquired immunity and autoimmune disease. Frontiers in immunology. 2018 Oct 4;9:2279.

10. Feldman CH, Malspeis S, Leatherwood C, Kubzansky L, Costenbader KH, Roberts AL. Association of childhood abuse with incident systemic lupus erythematosus in adulthood in a longitudinal cohort of women. The Journal of rheumatology. 2019 Dec 1;46(12):1589-96.

11. Cal SF. Depression and Systemic Lupus Erythematosus: A Case Report.

12. He Y, Sawalha AH. Drug-induced lupus erythematosus: an update on drugs and mechanisms. Current opinion in rheumatology. 2018 Sep;30(5):490.

13. Gryka-Marton M, Szukiewicz D, Teliga-Czajkowska J, Olesinska M. An overview of neonatal lupus with anti-Ro characteristics. International Journal of Molecular Sciences. 2021 Jan;22(17):9281.

14. Fava A, Petri M. Systemic lupus erythematosus: diagnosis and clinical management. Journal of autoimmunity. 2019 Jan 1;96:1-3.

15. Sloan M, Harwood R, Sutton S, D'Cruz D, Howard P, Wincup C, Brimicombe J, Gordon C. Medically explained symptoms: a mixed methods study of diagnostic, symptom and support experiences of patients with lupus and related systemic autoimmune diseases. Rheumatology advances in practice. 2020;4(1):rkaa006.

16. Saletra A, Olesi̇lska M. Quality of life in systemic lupus erythematosus and its measurement. Reumatologia/Rheumatology. 2018;56(1):45-54.

17. Aljaberi N, Bennett M, Brunner HI, Devarajan P. Proteomic profiling of urine: implications for lupus nephritis. Expert review of proteomics. 2019 Apr 3;16(4):303-13.

18. Ayoub I, Cassol C, Almaani S, Rovin B, Parikh SV. The kidney biopsy in systemic lupus erythematosus: a view of the past and a vision of the future. Advances in chronic kidney disease. 2019 Sep 1;26(5):360-8.

19. Pejchinovski M, Siwy J, Mullen W, Mischak H, Petri MA, Burkly LC, Wei R. Urine peptidomic biomarkers for diagnosis of patients with systematic lupus erythematosus. Lupus. 2018 Jan;27(1):6-16.

20. Parikh SV, Almaani S, Brodsky S, Rovin BH. Update on lupus nephritis: core curriculum 2020. American Journal of Kidney Diseases. 2020 Aug 1;76(2):265-81.

21. Barber MR, Drenkard C, Falasinnu T, Hoi A, Mak A, Kow NY, Svenungsson E, Peterson J, Clarke AE, Ramsey-Goldman R. Global epidemiology of systemic lupus erythematosus. Nature Reviews Rheumatology. 2021 Sep;17(9):515-32.

22. Bertoli A, López Pérez MJ, Alba P, Albiero A, Albiero E, Alessio D. Cumulative Rate and Factors Associated with Self-Reported Work Disability among Patients with Systemic Lupus Erythematosus: Data from the Province of Cordoba, Argentina. Clin Case Rep Int. 2022; 6.;1304.

23. Kusnanto K, Sari NP, Harmayetty H, Efendi F, Gunawan J. Self-care model application to improve self-care agency, self-care activities, and quality of life in patients with systemic lupus erythematosus. Journal of Taibah University medical sciences. 2018 Oct 1;13(5):472-8.

24. Izmirly PM, Parton H, Wang L, McCune WJ, Lim SS, Drenkard C, Ferucci ED, Dall'Era M, Gordon C, Helmick CG, Somers EC. Prevalence of Systemic Lupus Erythematosus in the United States: Estimates From a Meta□Analysis of the Centers for Disease Control and Prevention National Lupus Registries. Arthritis & Rheumatology. 2021 Jun;73(6):991-6.

25. Pons-Estel GJ, Ugarte-Gil MF, Alarcón GS. Epidemiology of systemic lupus erythematosus. Expert review of clinical immunology. 2017 Aug 3;13(8):799-814.

26. https://www.lupus.org/news/healthcare-costs-rise-as-lupus-disease-activity-increases

27. Leuchten N, Milke B, Winkler-Rohlfing B, Daikh D, Dörner T, Johnson SR, Aringer M. Early symptoms of systemic lupus erythematosus (SLE) recalled by 339 SLE patients. Lupus. 2018 Aug;27(9):1431-6.

28. Souza RR, Barreto MD, Teston EF, Reis PD, Cecilio HP, Marcon SS. Duality Of Living With Systemic Lupus Erythematosus: Fluctuating Between "Good Days" And "Bad Days." Texto & Contexto-Enfermagem. 2021 Aug 2;30.

29. Elera-Fitzcarrald C, Fuentes A, González LA, Burgos PI, Alarcón GS, Ugarte-Gil MF. Factors affecting quality of life in patients with systemic lupus erythematosus: important considerations and potential interventions. Expert Review of Clinical Immunology. 2018 Nov 2;14(11):915-31.

30. Mason A, Anver H, Lwin M, Holroyd C, Faust SN, Edwards CJ. Lupus, vaccinations and COVID-19: what we know now. Lupus. 2021 Sep;30(10):1541-52.

31. Wen L, Labopin M, Badoglio M, Wang D, Sun L, Farge-Bancel D. Prognostic factors for clinical response in systemic lupus erythematosus patients treated by allogeneic mesenchymal stem cells. Stem Cells International. 2019 May 2;2019.

32. Deeks ED. Anifrolumab: first approval. Drugs. 2021 Oct;81(15):1795-802.

33. Vital EM, Merrill JT, Morand EF, Furie RA, Bruce IN, Tanaka Y, Manzi S, Kalunian KC, Kalyani RN, Streicher K, Abreu G. Anifrolumab efficacy and safety by type I interferon gene signature and clinical subgroups in patients with SLE: post hoc analysis of pooled data from two phase III trials. Annals of the rheumatic diseases. 2022 Jul 1;81(7):951-61.

34. https://expertscape.com/ex/lupus+erythematosus%2C+systemic/p/earth

35. https://kaleidoscopefightinglupus.org/alternative-lupus-treat-ments-and-therapies/

36. Jesus D, Rodrigues M, Matos A, Henriques C, Pereira da Silva JA, Inês LS. Performance of SLEDAI-2K to detect a clinically meaning-ful change in SLE disease activity: a 36-month prospective cohort study of 334 patients. Lupus. 2019 Apr;28(5):607-12.

37. Thanou A, Jupe E, Purushothaman M, Niewold TB, Munroe ME. Clinical disease activity and flare in SLE: Current concepts and novel biomarkers. Journal of Autoimmunity. 2021 May 1;119:102615.

38. https://www.ranker.com/list/famous-people-with-lupus/celeb-rity-lists

39. Kono M, Nagafuchi Y, Shoda H, Fujio K. The impact of obesity and a high-fat diet on clinical and immunological features in systemic lupus erythematosus. Nutrients. 2021 Feb 4;13(2):504.

40. https://www.lupus.org/sites/default/files/media/docu-ments/2020-2021-LFA_Annual_Report_0.pdft

41. https://www.lupusresearch.org/who-we-are/about-lupus-re-search-alliance/financials/

42. https://worldlupusfederation.org/our-mission/

43. https://www.hopkinslupus.org/lupus-treatment/lupus-medica-tions/dhea/

NOTES

NOTES

NOTES

NOTES

Visit **www.starvingthewolf.com**
and subscribe to receive exclusive updates.

You'll have early access to
new content, events, and projects
that expand on the insights shared in this book.

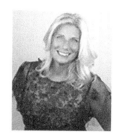 **Karen Quiros** is a dedicated holistic wellness practitioner and the visionary behind Balanced Wellness Consulting. Her life's work is deeply rooted in the pursuit of holistic health and personal transformation. Her unwavering dedication to healing, personal development, and enhancing the well-being of others inspires and leads many on their journey toward wellness.

Nearly four decades ago, Karen embarked on her holistic wellness journey, driven by the need for alternative treatments to conventional methods for lupus and endometriosis. This quest led her to master health coaching, nutrition, positive psychology, energy and sound healing, quantum biofeedback, and herbal medicine. Recognizing the vital role of movement, mindfulness, and spiritual growth in healing, Karen obtained certifications in meditation, yoga, and personal training. Her holistic approach is further enriched by her participation in transformative programs like Chakradance® and SoulCollage®.

The pinnacle of Karen's holistic wellness practice is her innovative Happiness Compass© program, a testament to her comprehensive approach to healing and personal growth. Ingeniously crafted, this program guides participants on a transformative journey, employing self-awareness, exploration, guided visualization, and creativity, unveiling their unique paths toward healing, happiness, and life purpose. This workshop epitomizes Karen's dedication to fostering profound personal change and embodies the essence of her work in holistic wellness.

A native of Long Island, Karen's personal life is as rich and fulfilling as her professional endeavors. She celebrates a 30-year marriage and is the proud mother of two extraordinary sons. Embracing a homesteader lifestyle, she is deeply connected to nature, engaging in gardening, beekeeping, and caring for chickens. Her hobbies, which include travel, baking, knitting, yoga, cycling, and embarking on hiking adventures, reflect her commitment to a well-balanced and holistic lifestyle.

Made in United States
North Haven, CT
12 November 2024